EMBRYO CLEAVAGE

胚胎分裂

（美）武彬（Bin Wu）编著

吴方贵 刘尚杰 郑洲 张敏旗 译

中山大学出版社
·广州·

Chinese Translation© 2021 Wu Fanggui, Liu Shangjie, Zheng Zhou, Zhang Minqi, Sun-Yat-Sen University Press
Translation from the English Edition
Copyright 2017 Bin Wu and the authors
All Rights Reserved

版权所有　翻印必究

图书在版编目（CIP）数据

胚胎分裂/（美）武彬（Bin Wu）编著；吴方贵等译. —广州：中山大学出版社，2022.12
书名原文：Embryo Cleavage
ISBN 978-7-306-07635-9

Ⅰ.①胚…　Ⅱ.①武…②吴…　Ⅲ.①人体胚胎学　Ⅳ.①R321

中国版本图书馆 CIP 数据核字（2022）第 207660 号

出 版 人：王天琪
策划编辑：鲁佳慧
责任编辑：鲁佳慧
封面设计：曾　斌
责任校对：麦颖晖
责任技编：靳晓虹
出版发行：中山大学出版社
电　　话：编辑部 020-84110283，84113349，84111997，84110779，84110776
　　　　　发行部 020-84111998，84111981，84111160
地　　址：广州市新港西路 135 号
邮　　编：510275　　传　　真：020-84036565
网　　址：http://www.zsup.com.cn　E-mail：zdcbs@mail.sysu.edu.cn
印 刷 者：恒美印务（广州）有限公司
规　　格：787mm×1092mm　1/16　6.625 印张　158 千字
版次印次：2022 年 12 月第 1 版　2022 年 12 月第 1 次印刷
定　　价：65.00 元

如发现本书因印装质量影响阅读，请与出版社发行部联系调换

· 原著作者简介 ·

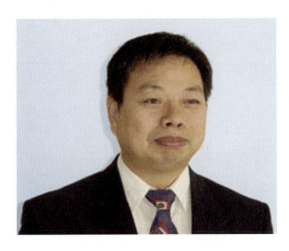

武 彬 博士，美国生物分析学会（American Board of Bioanalysis，ABB）授予的高精复杂临床实验室主任（High Complexity Clinical Laboratory Director，HCLD），美国亚利桑那州生殖医学研究中心试管婴儿实验室主任，美国生殖医学学会、国际胚胎移植学会、生殖生物学学会、美国生物分析学会及欧洲人类生殖和胚胎学会的会员。在中国西北农业大学（现西北农林科技大学）获得学士、硕士和博士学位。1990年率先在国内从事动物血液蛋白质多态性的遗传标记研究。1992年后在美国爱达荷大学、美国康奈尔大学和加拿大圭尔夫大学进行博士后工作，着重进行动物配子发生和胚胎发育的分子机制研究，在国际杂志上率先发表《c-Mos原癌蛋白在牛卵母细胞成熟中的调节作用》。1994年在澳大利亚国际胚胎移植会议上获得研究报告二等奖。1998年被西北农业大学评为教授、博士研究生导师。1999年起于美国芝加哥从事人类胚胎生物工程——试管婴儿的研究和生产工作。曾于SCI国际杂志以及国际学术会议上发表论文和作报告30多篇/次，并获奖4项。近20年来主要从事人类试管婴儿的研究和临床工作，卵子和胚胎的发育机制及精子、卵子和胚胎的遗传学诊断研究。2014年7月被美国胚胎学家学会授予"杰出胚胎学家"荣誉称号。

· 译者简介 ·

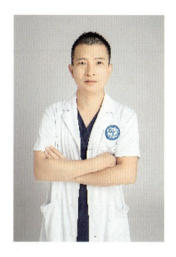

吴方贵 广东省临床医学会生殖医学专业委员会青年委员，广东省泌尿生殖协会检验医学分会委员，广东省医疗行业协会生殖医学管理分会委员。就职于深圳市罗湖区人民医院生殖医学科。一直从事生殖胚胎实验室及分子遗传工作，具有娴熟的胚胎实验室技能和丰富的实验室管理水平，擅长胚胎培养技术、胚胎选择、实验室质量控制、实验室流程化及信息化管理。主持和参与了多项实验室技术平台构建，作为项目主要负责人参与科研立项10多项，获软件著作权2项，获专利10多项，发表论文多篇。

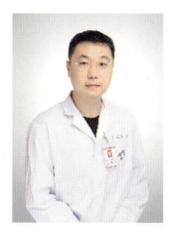

刘尚杰 博士，副研究员，硕士研究生导师，中国科学院广州生物医药与健康研究院细胞生物学方向博士后，就职于深圳市罗湖区人民医院生殖医学科。广东省医学会生殖医学分会基础研究学组成员，广东省临床医学学会生殖医学专业委员会青年委员，广东省医疗行业协会生殖医学管理分会委员，深圳市高层次专业人才，罗湖区高层次医疗人才。2013年开始从事辅助生殖胚胎实验室及分子遗传工作。主持并参与多个科研项目，主持国家级项目2项，省部级项目1项，参与完成2项省级应用技术科技成果。在国内外学术刊物上发表论文多篇，其中以第一作者在 *Cell Biology and Toxicology Molecules* 等杂志上发表SCI论文5篇。申请专利5项，已授权发明专利2项、实用新型专利3项。

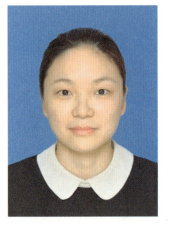

郑　洲　博士，助理研究员，广州医科大学临床检验学方向博士后，深圳市罗湖医院集团临床医学检验中心科研骨干。现主要从事临床医学检验及生殖医学相关研究。作为主要工作者参与多项国家级研究课题，目前以第一作者在 *Virulence* 等国际期刊上发表 SCI 论文 8 篇。

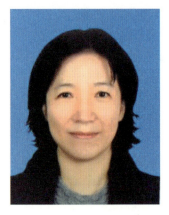

张敏旗　主任医师，深圳市罗湖区人民医院生殖医学科主任。广东省临床医学会生殖医学分会委员，广东省生殖免疫与内分泌专科联盟理事，深圳市医学会生殖医学专业委员会委员。从事生殖妇产临床工作 20 多年，具有扎实的妇产科理论基础和较为丰富的妇产科、生殖医学临床和实验研究技能。主持并参与多个省、市级研究项目，在国内外学术刊物上发表论文多篇，出版专著 1 部。申请授权实用新型专利 4 项。

Preface for *Embryo Cleavage*

Embryo cleavage is the division of cells in the early embryo. This division from one celled zygote into 2 cells, 4 cells, 8 cells and 16 cells, morula stage and final forming blastocyst stage until implanting in the uterus is called embryo cleavage. These stage embryos still do not implant in the uterus and also they are called as preimplantation embryos. Preimplantation embryo development experiences a series of critical events and remarkable epigenetic modifications and reprogramming of gene expression occurs to activate the embryonic genome. The development of current assisted reproductive technology (ART) has created some new observations and novel discoveries in cleavage embryos. For example, in order to observe embryo morphology and assess embryo quality, time-lapse imaging and light-sheet microscopy have made it possible to visualize early mammalian development in greater detail and over longer time periods than ever before. Thus, this book will collect some new technologies and methods on the study of cleavage embryos to select high quality embryos for transfer and improve embryo implantation and pregnancy.

Since the birth of the first in vitro fertilization (IVF or test-tube) baby, ART has been widely used in human infertility treatment and animal population reproduction and expansion. However, the success of assisted reproductive technology mainly depends on the production of viable embryos with high implantation potential. More importantly, choosing the best embryo for transfer has become the major challenge in IVF. In the early embryo culture, the embryo quality assessment was mainly based on the morphological criteria of transfer embryo. Thus, performing serial observation of embryo morphology is a common technique for embryologists to evaluate embryos and has been considered as key predictor of implantation and pregnancy. For a long term, embryologists perform embryo quality and morphology assessment by taking embryos out of incubator and placing under a microscope. However, although this is easily practice, it frequently takes embryos out of incubator which dues to concerns for safety and stability of culture conditions. Also, some key points of embryonic development may be missed for observation. Recently, various time-lapse microscopy incubators have started to be used in human IVF clinic to monitor all step of embryo growth and development. Time-lapse imaging is another non-invasive, emerging technology that allows 24-hour monitoring of embryo development, offering the possibility of increased quantity and quality of morphological information without disturbing the culture condition. This technique has been able to improve transferred embryo implantation and pregnancy. Thus, in the second part of this book, some morphokinetic markers

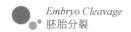

can be revealed in time-lapse system. The first is the time outline of embryo cleavage and embryologists may clearly know what situation embryo should be at various time points. Thus, an optimal quality embryo or high potential implantation embryo may be selected for transfer to obtain a higher pregnancy rate. Secondly, some specific events (such as a four dimensional video sequencing of embryos) of cleavage embryos may be observed by morphokinetic markers and spatio-temporal analysis and innovated computer hardware and software analysis to determine embryo developmental speed, sex, etc. Simultaneous monitoring of molecular processes enables the study of connections between genetic expression and cell physiology and development.

Cleavage embryos experiences a series of gene expression. In the early stages, maternal mRNAs direct embryonic development. New study showed that differential demethylation process resultsin differential parental gene expression in the early developing embryos that may have an impact on the correct development. Thus, Part III lists a review paper which showed different factors affecting gene expression during early embryo development, which includes epigenetic factors, focusing on methylation profiles. The effects of noncoding RNAs on gene expression were thoroughly evaluated. Based on the products of gene expression, an available metabolic and proteomic approaches as the non-invasive molecular assessment of embryo viability has been described. A new discovery, the alpha-1 chain of the human haptoglobin molecule may be as a quantitative biomarker of embryo viability. If this molecular composition of cultivation media can be used as an additional non-invasive procedure to choose an embryo for selective transfer, it will be very useful to improve human IVF pregnancy outcome.

Embryonic quality, cleavage speed, gene expression have a close relationship with in vitro culture environment, including culture media, incubator type, gas concentration. Thus, an optimum for embryo in vitro culture plays important rules in improving embryo quality and pregnancy rate. In the last part of this book, an interesting research report has been listed, in which showed the favorable response of individual patient's embryos to media and incubators. Some patents' embryos grow very well in one kind of medium, but it doesn't grow well in the other medium. Thus, in human IVF clinic practice, using two media and two incubators for embryo culture could significantly improve IVF/ICSI embryo quality and increase pregnant rates.

Great thanks go to all authors who gladly contributed their time and expertise to prepare these outstanding chapters included in this book.

Bin Wu, Ph. D., HCLD (ABB)
Arizona Center for Reproductive Endocrinology and Infertility
Tucson, Arizona
USA

原 著 序

　　胚胎分裂是指早期胚胎的细胞分裂，即从单细胞受精卵分裂为 2 个、4 个、8 个和 16 个细胞，并经历桑葚胚期、囊胚期，直至植入子宫前，整个过程称为胚胎分裂。这些阶段的胚胎还没有被植入子宫，因此也称为植入前胚胎。胚胎分裂经历了一系列关键事件后，发生了显著的表观遗传修饰和基因表达重编程，以激活胚胎基因组。随着辅助生殖技术的发展，在卵裂胚胎的研究和临床实践中出现了一些新的观察方法和新的发现。例如，通过光学显微镜观察早期胚胎，并对其进行更详细的观察，可能获得更长的胚胎发育时间和更高的胚胎发育质量。因此，本书收集了一些关于胚胎分裂研究的新技术和新方法，以选择高质量的胚胎进行移植，并改善胚胎种植率和妊娠率。

　　自首例试管婴儿诞生以来，人类辅助生殖技术已被广泛应用于治疗不孕症。然而，辅助生殖技术的成功主要取决于具有高着床潜能的活胚胎。更重要的是，选择最佳的胚胎进行移植已经成为体外受精的主要挑战。在早期胚胎培养中，胚胎质量评估主要基于移植胚胎的形态学标准。因此，对胚胎形态进行连续观察是胚胎学家评估胚胎的常用技术，并被认为是胚胎着床和妊娠的关键预测因素。长期以来，胚胎学家通过将胚胎从培养箱中取出并放在显微镜下进行胚胎质量和形态评估，尽管这很容易实施，但频繁将胚胎从培养箱中取出会影响培养条件的安全性和稳定性。此外，胚胎发育的一些关键点可能会被忽略。近年来，各种时差显微镜培养箱开始在人类体外受精临床上用于监测胚胎生长发育的各个阶段。时差成像是另一种无创的新兴技术，允许 24 h 监测胚胎发育，提供在不干扰培养条件的情况下提高形态学信息数量和质量的可能性。这项技术已经能够改善移植胚胎的种植率和妊娠率。因此，在本书第 2 章，一些形态动力学标记可以在时间推移系统中被揭示。首先是胚胎分裂的时间轮廓，胚胎学家可以清楚地知道胚胎在不同时间点的情况，因此，可以选择最佳质量的胚胎或高植入潜能的胚胎进行移植，以获得更高的妊娠率。其次，通过形态动力学标记和时空分析以及创新的计算机硬件和软件分析，可以观察到胚胎分裂的一些特定事件（如胚胎的四维视频分析），以确定胚胎发育速度和性别等其他信息。同时，监测胚胎分裂的分子过程，可以深入研究基因表达与细胞生理和发育之间的联系。

　　胚胎分裂经历了一系列的基因表达变迁过程。在早期阶段，母体 mRNAs 指导胚胎发育。新的研究表明，不同的去甲基化过程导致早期发育胚胎中不同的亲本基因表达，这可能会影响正常的发育。因此，本书第 3 章展示了早期胚胎发育过程中影响基因表达的不同因素，包括表观遗传因素（重点关注甲基化谱）。同时，针对非编码 RNA 对基因表达的影响也进行了全面评估。基于基因表达产物，描述了一种可用的代谢和蛋白质组学方法，作为胚胎存活的无创分子评估的手段。一项新的研究结果表明，人类结合珠蛋

白分子的 α-1 链可能是胚胎活力的定量生物标志物。如果这种培养基的分子组成可以作为一种额外的无创程序来选择胚胎以进行选择性移植，它将对改善人类体外受精妊娠结局非常有用。

胚胎质量、分裂速度、基因表达与体外培养环境（包括培养基、培养箱类型及气体浓度）密切相关。因此，胚胎体外培养的最佳条件对提高胚胎质量和妊娠率具有重要意义。本书最后一章介绍了患者的胚胎对培养基和培养箱的选择性，如一些患者的胚胎在一种培养基中生长良好，但在另一种培养基中生长欠佳。因此，在人类体外受精临床实践中，使用两种不同类型的培养基和两种不同款型的培养箱进行胚胎培养可以显著提高体外受精或卵胞质内单精子注射胚胎的质量和妊娠率。

非常感谢所有乐意贡献时间和专业知识来准备本书的杰出作者们。

武彬博士，HCLD（ABB）
亚利桑那生殖内分泌与不孕症中心
美国，亚利桑那州，图森

序

　　这是一本关于人类辅助生殖技术胚胎实验室业务新进展的论著。在英文原作者武彬先生的帮助和指导下，深圳市罗湖区人民医院的吴方贵、刘尚杰两位胚胎学家共同组织完成了翻译工作。6年前，译者吴方贵曾在北京大学第三医院生殖医学中心的胚胎实验室进修，他留给大家的印象是稳重、谦和、有责任心。无论是在进修期间还是返回原单位后，他对学习专业新知识和新技能都非常积极，始终与我们实验室保持着业务联系和学术交流。

　　20世纪70年代末，世界上第一个体外受精-胚胎移植技术妊娠分娩的婴儿诞生，至今"试管婴儿"已达数百万个。人类胚胎实验室技术的快速发展吸引了大量的专业技术人员加入这个行业。体外受精-胚胎移植技术的发展，不仅为广大不孕不育夫妇提供了独特的医疗手段，而且为研究探索人类着床前胚胎发育的形态动力学及分子事件提供了观察窗口，让我们在认识着床前胚胎发育特点的同时，还有可能获得解决一些临床问题的契机和手段。目前，体外受精-胚胎移植治疗的活产率在40%左右，还有提升空间。胚胎实验室技术人员在完成常规技术操作的同时，迫切需要更深入地了解胚胎发育的规律，更准确地进行胚胎质量评价，更充分地营造适合胚胎体外生长发育的培养体系。

　　本书共7章，按照胚胎发育过程的时间轴展开，论述了从受精卵到卵裂期胚胎的形态学特点，介绍了利用时差成像观察到的胚胎发育的特殊时间节点，以及如何采用培养胚胎后的液体进行检测、评估胚胎发育潜能等。此外，本书还包括如何选择培养液和培养箱以提高培养效果等内容。本书的特点是利用较先进的技术手段，研究胚胎形态和形态动力学及基因表达特点，呈现胚胎发育的生理过程，认识胚胎发育过程中的分子事件。本书内容是近年来本研究领域的前沿进展，对胚胎实验室技术人员和生殖临床医生有很好的参考价值，能帮助大家更好地认识受精卵及胚胎发育。

　　本人非常高兴看到这样一部有学术价值的专著能被翔实准确地翻译成中文。译者在临床工作之余，完成了大量的翻译工作，为大家呈上了一部准确、易读的中文译著，便于国内广大生殖医学实验室和临床工作人员阅读学习，提升专业水平，更好地为患者服务。

北京大学第三医院生殖医学中心
2023年3月

前　言

我国人口规模较大，相应的育龄人口基数庞大。资料显示，不孕症发病率为5%～15%，人类辅助生殖技术的广泛应用给众多不孕症患者带来生育希望。体外授精-胚胎移植技术是非常有效的辅助生殖技术之一。历经40多年的研究积累、临床实践，人类辅助生殖技术已在全世界范围广泛使用，新的生殖医学理论与技术飞速发展，不断更新。

深圳市罗湖区人民医院（深圳大学第三附属医院）生殖医学科成立于1998年2月，是深圳市卫生系统第一家开展辅助生育技术的生殖医学中心，深圳市首例体外受精-胚胎移植试管婴儿、卵胞质内单精子注射试管婴儿、胚胎种植前遗传学诊断试管婴儿均诞生于本科室。2017年，美国亚利桑那生殖医学研究中心试管婴儿实验室主任武彬教授前来本生殖医学科参观指导，我们有幸认识了武彬教授。而后我们在Intech Open阅读到武彬教授的著作 *Embryo Cleavage*，收获颇丰。

原著从胚胎分裂时间轴、胚胎时差成像研究、胚胎分裂时空分析、胚胎基因表达与表观遗传学控制、基于分析培养液的胚胎无创评估、不同类型培养基的影响等方面进行了详细阐述，收集了关于胚胎研究的新技术和新方法，用以选择高质量的胚胎进行移植，进而改善胚胎着床和妊娠状况。本书对于辅助生殖从业人员、胚胎学家及科研人员了解胚胎发育及胚胎选择，是一本非常有价值的参考书。

为让更多同行从中获益，我们组织人员对该书进行了中文翻译。非常有幸，我们的翻译工作得到了原著作者武彬教授的大力支持和帮助，感谢武彬教授给予的指导及审校。我们希望本译著的出版，在普及胚胎发育相关知识的同时，能让更多的辅助生殖从业人员了解及提升相应的专业技能，从而使患者获益。

在此，我们对原著作者武彬教授与原著中的其他作者，以及为我们的翻译工作提供帮助的所有人员，表示衷心的感谢。由于译者水平有限，本译著可能存在一些不妥或错误之处，恳请国内外同道和广大读者批评指正。

深圳市罗湖区人民医院（深圳大学第三附属医院）生殖医学科
吴方贵　刘尚杰
2022年3月

目　录

第1章　胚胎分裂研究的新技术 ·· 1
　1　从受精卵到卵裂期胚胎的观察 ·· 1
　　　1.1　基于时差成像的胚胎分裂形态动力学 ··· 4
　　　1.2　通过培养基分析对卵裂期胚胎的基因表达及发育潜能进行无创评估 ······ 5
　2　改善胚胎分裂的体外培养环境 ·· 6
　　参考文献 ·· 6

第2章　胚胎分裂时间轴 ·· 10
　1　形态学标记 ··· 10
　2　时差成像中的特殊标记 ··· 13
　3　结论 ·· 14
　　参考文献 ·· 14

第3章　基于时差成像观测的胚胎形态动力学研究 ·· 16
　1　时差成像 ·· 17
　　　1.1　时差形态动力学参数和胚胎着床潜能 ··· 17
　　　1.2　性别对胚胎形态动力学的影响 ·· 19
　　　1.3　碎片对胚胎形态动力学的影响 ·· 19
　　　1.4　卵巢刺激方案对胚胎形态动力学的影响 ··· 19
　　　1.5　培养基类型对胚胎形态动力学的影响 ··· 20
　　　1.6　用于预测胚胎着床潜能的形态动力学算法 ··· 20
　　　1.7　基于时差成像观察的不同研究 ·· 22
　　　1.8　结论 ··· 22
　　参考文献 ·· 23

第4章 体外胚胎分裂的时空分析方法 ·········· 29
- 1 活体成像在胚胎学中的作用 ·········· 30
- 2 胚胎成像的无创技术 ·········· 30
  - 2.1 荧光成像 ·········· 31
  - 2.2 无标记显微镜 ·········· 31
- 3 活胚胎成像的挑战 ·········· 32
- 4 方法1：使用荧光标记的三维小鼠胚胎形态 ·········· 34
- 5 方法2：使用机器学习对人类胚胎进行细胞谱系研究 ·········· 35
- 6 方法3：使用视频图像处理的人类胚胎分析 ·········· 37
- 7 结论 ·········· 41
- 参考文献 ·········· 41

第5章 胚胎基因表达和表观遗传学的控制 ·········· 48
- 1 基因表达与表观遗传学 ·········· 49
  - 1.1 合子和着床前胚胎的表观遗传修饰 ·········· 49
  - 1.2 配子的表观遗传修饰 ·········· 50
- 2 基因表达和短链非编码RNA：miRNA ·········· 51
  - 2.1 miRNA生物发生 ·········· 51
  - 2.2 miRNA在着床前胚胎中的表达 ·········· 52
- 3 基因表达与长链非编码RNA ·········· 53
- 4 基因表达与人类辅助生殖技术 ·········· 54
- 5 结论 ·········· 54
- 参考文献 ·········· 54

第6章 通过分析培养基对胚胎存活率进行无创评估 ·········· 64
- 1 胚胎形态学 ·········· 65
- 2 胚胎培养基的分析 ·········· 66
- 3 代谢组学研究 ·········· 67
- 4 蛋白质组学研究 ·········· 68
- 5 使用结合珠蛋白α-1链的定量测定评估胚胎生存能力 ·········· 70
- 6 胚胎早期发育中的细胞凋亡 ·········· 71
- 7 结论 ·········· 72

参考文献 …………………………………………………………………………… 73

第7章　两种不同类型培养基和两种不同款型培养箱协同作用改善辅助生殖技术妊娠结局 …………………………………………………………………………… 76
　　1　材料和方法 ………………………………………………………………………… 77
　　　　1.1　培养基 ……………………………………………………………………… 77
　　　　1.2　培养箱 ……………………………………………………………………… 77
　　2　实验设计 …………………………………………………………………………… 78
　　3　结果 ………………………………………………………………………………… 79
　　　　3.1　新发现 ……………………………………………………………………… 79
　　　　3.2　实验验证 …………………………………………………………………… 80
　　4　讨论 ………………………………………………………………………………… 85
　　5　结论 ………………………………………………………………………………… 86
　　参考文献 ……………………………………………………………………………… 87

第1章 胚胎分裂研究的新技术

哺乳动物的精子与卵细胞结合受精后形成胚胎，胚胎形成是指胚胎发育早期阶段发生的细胞分裂和分化的过程。在胚胎学中，胚胎分裂是指早期胚胎的细胞分裂，即单细胞受精卵从1个细胞分裂成2个、4个、8个和16个细胞，并经历桑葚胚期、囊胚期，直至植入子宫前，整个过程称为胚胎分裂。许多物种的受精卵经历了快速的细胞周期，并没有明显的体积增长，形成与原始受精卵大小相同的细胞群。分裂过程中产生的不同细胞称为卵裂球，其随着胚胎发育逐步形成一个紧凑的团块，称为桑葚胚。胚胎分裂以囊胚的形成而结束，该阶段胚胎也称为着床前胚胎。

在过去的30年里，随着人类辅助生殖技术（assisted reproductive technology，ART）的发展，针对植入前胚胎研究，特别是在胚胎分裂过程中，有了一些新的观察结果和发现。植入前胚胎发育经历了一系列的关键事件和显著的表观遗传学修饰，基因表达的重新编程激活了胚胎的基因组。这些事件的改变往往会导致胚胎质量和形态的改变。在胚胎分裂阶段，虽然传统的标准形态学评估与染色体异常关系不大[1]，但形态学评估依然是评估胚胎质量的一个主要工具。因此，目前已发展出许多新的观察方法和技术。例如，为了观察胚胎形态和评估胚胎质量，时差成像和光片照明显微镜的使用，使我们有可能比以往任何时候都更详细和在更长的时间内观察哺乳动物胚胎的早期发育状况[2-4]。本书收集了一些关于卵裂期胚胎研究的新技术和方法，用以选择高质量的胚胎进行移植，进而改善胚胎着床和妊娠情况。

1 从受精卵到卵裂期胚胎的观察

1912年报道了第一例兔胚胎培养[5]和小鼠受精卵在体外培养形成囊胚的[6-7]相关研究，发现胚胎质量与胚胎在子宫内着床密切相关，胚胎质量是体外胚胎移植到子宫后影响妊娠的重要因素之一。自1978年7月第一例试管婴儿路易丝-布朗出生，胚胎体外培育（in vitro embryo production，IVEP）已被广泛用于人类不孕症治疗以及动物群体的繁殖和扩大。2010年诺贝尔生理学或医学奖授予罗伯特-爱德华兹，以表彰他开发体外受精胚胎移植技术（in vitro fertilization and embryo transfer，IVF-ET）用于治疗非输卵管因素妇女的不孕症。然而，人类 ART 的成功主要取决于获得具有高着床潜能的胚胎。更重要的是，选择最佳的胚胎进行移植已成为体外受精（in vitro fertilization，IVF）的主要挑战。在早期的胚胎培养中，胚胎质量的评估主要是基于移植胚胎的形态学标准。因此，进行胚胎形态的连续观察是胚胎学家评估胚胎质量的常用技术，也被认为是预测着床和妊娠的关键因素[8-10]。长期以来，胚胎学家都是将胚胎从培养箱中取出，并放在显微镜下进行胚胎质量和形态学评估。除了形态学观察，研究人员也对细胞核变化、基因激活和表达、胞质蛋白表达、胚胎分化等方面进行了一系列研究。然而，这些研究往往会导致胚胎的死亡。例如，在早期的研究中，观察精子进入卵子或激活卵细胞后的微纺锤体变化，需要将受精卵或激活的卵子固定在玻片上，用免疫细胞化学荧光素进行染色，再用激光扫描共聚焦显微镜观察[11]。我们的研究清楚地显示了牛卵母细胞激活和卵胞质内单精子注射（intracytoplasmic sperm injection，ICSI）后纺锤体及染色质

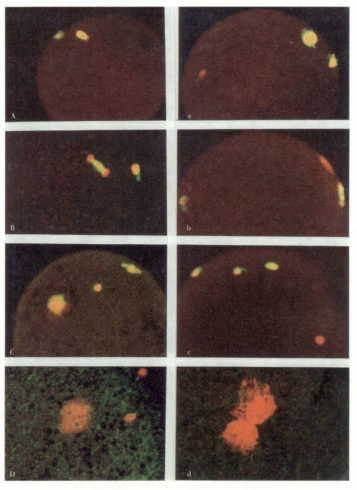

大写字母表示激活后的变化，小写字母表示 ICSI 后的变化。A/a 显示为激活后 0.5 h，B/b 为激活后 2 h，C/c 为激活后 3 h，D/d 为激活后 7 h 或 ICSI 后。激活卵中的原核和 ICSI 卵中的原核呈现红色。

图 1-1 激光扫描共聚焦显微镜观察牛卵母细胞激活和卵胞质内单精子注射（ICSI）后不同时间点的纺锤体和染色质变化

的改变（图1-1）。精子进入卵母细胞，或钙离子、乙醇都可能激活卵母细胞并导致第二极体的排出。为了观察第二极体出现的时间，我们对激活后各阶段的卵母细胞进行染色，结果显示，激活后5 h，第二极体可能完全被排出（图1-2）。

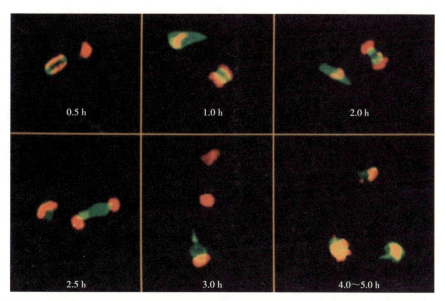

激活后0.5 h，纺锤体与染色体开始分裂，完成纺锤体分裂需要约3 h，第二极体可能在激活后约5 h被排出。红色和绿色一起表示纺锤体，红色点表示第一极体。

图1-2　激光扫描共聚焦显微镜观察牛卵母细胞激活后不同时间的纺锤体与染色质变化

基因表达的研究往往需要从胚胎中分离出mRNA或蛋白质[12-14]，因此，胚胎需要被裂解，这会让胚胎失活。而研究桑葚期和囊胚期胚胎的细胞分化，常用荧光素双染色显微观察的方法来区分内细胞团（inner cell mass，ICM）和滋养外胚层（trophectoderm，TE），根据不同的颜色（ICM为蓝色，TE为粉红色，图1-3）来计算两种细胞的数量。

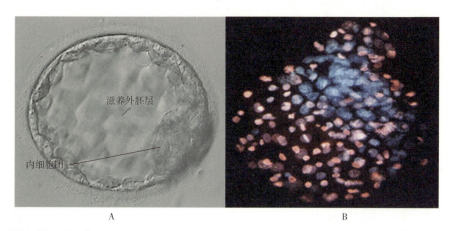

A. 显微镜明场下囊胚期胚胎，具有明显的ICM和TE。B. 双染牛囊胚胚胎，蓝色为ICM，粉色为TE（感谢杜富良教授提供图片）。

图1-3　用双荧光染色法鉴别牛囊胚中的不同细胞

上述这些研究方法都会损害胚胎，因此不可能将这些方法应用于临床实践中。目前的胚胎质量评估主要是基于移植胚胎的形态学标准，其中，卵裂球均一性、碎片和细胞质颗粒程度3个参数成为主要形态学评估指标[15]。同时，不同培养日的胚胎细胞数和多核性也可以用来评估胚胎质量[16-17]。一些研究报告记录了卵裂期胚胎的形态特征与妊娠率之间的联系。因此，形态学评估是目前人类体外受精和动物体外胚胎培育中评估胚胎质量的基本方法。然而，尽管该方法很容易实行，但需要经常将胚胎移出培养箱，这可能对培养条件的安全性和稳定性产生影响[18]。此外，间断的观察过程可能会使观察者错过胚胎发育的一些关键节点。但整体而言，培养过程中和胚胎移植前对胚胎进行评估是一个重要的临床工作。目前，对体外受精胚胎的主要评估依然是使用显微镜进行观察。近年来，各种时差培养箱在人类IVF实验室中被用于监测胚胎生长和发育的所有过程。尽管胚胎植入前遗传学诊断（preimplantation genetic diagnosis，PGD）/植入前遗传学筛查（preimplantation genetic screening，PGS）技术已被应用于人类胚胎选择的实践中，并可以提高妊娠率，但这些技术对胚胎来说是有创的。寻找一种无创的方法来选择优质胚胎在人类ART实践中非常重要。Sallam等[19]回顾了无创的胚胎选择方法，并根据目前主要的证据对这些方法进行了评估，以期找出其中是否有成熟的方法可以取代或补充历史悠久的形态学评估方法。因此，我们需要更强大的工具来评估胚胎的形态动力学标记。

1.1　基于时差成像的胚胎分裂形态动力学

几十年来，研究人员一直试图跟踪从受精卵到成年个体的多细胞器官系统发育过程。虽然科学家们已经探索了这一过程的各个步骤，但不能实时模拟整个发育过程。最近，*Nature Methods* 杂志发表的2篇论文报道了光片照明显微镜的进展，使研究人员能够非常详细地观察胚胎的早期发育[3-4]。最新的光片照明显微镜使用激光照亮样品的一个薄片，并在一个快照中捕捉整个平面，这使其需要的光比共聚焦显微镜或双光子显微镜更少的光。使用该技术进行观察的速度非常快，也非常温和，在多个关键方面表现出色[20]。这种新的多视图成像技术能够很好地对果蝇、斑马鱼和小鼠的整个胚胎发育进行成像。

时差成像（time-lapse imaging，TLI）是另一种无创的新兴技术，可以24 h监测胚胎发育，提供了在不干扰培养条件的情况下增加形态学信息数量和质量的可能性[21]。时差显微镜对胚胎发育的观察非常有用。在过去的10年中，许多IVF中心已经使用时差成像技术监测体外培养过程中的胚胎生长和分裂，最后根据记录数据和图片来选择优质胚胎进行移植。据报道，这种技术能够改善移植胚胎的种植率和妊娠率[22-23]。根据胚胎分裂的时差记录，可以确定正常的胚胎分裂速度。因此，本书第2章利用时差成像，根据形态动力学标记，概述了胚胎分裂的时间。根据胚胎分裂时间，胚胎学家可以清楚地知道胚胎在不同的时间点应该处于发育的哪个阶段。基于此，应选择最佳质量或具有高着床潜能的胚胎进行移植，以获得更高的妊娠率。此外，时差成像可以揭示出一些形态动力学标记。例如，胚胎细胞在特定时间快速分裂往往会导致较低的种植率。在正常情况下，从受精卵分裂成2~3个细胞需要10~11 h。但Rubio等[21]发现，一些胚胎只用了约 5 h 就完成了这个过程，这些胚胎的种植率比正常分裂胚胎的低得多（1.2% vs 20.0%）。此外，胚胎不均等分裂是指 1 个胚胎分裂成 3 个子卵裂球，或细胞周期间隔少于 5 h，这往往会引起低种植率[24]。因此，我们可以使用这些更精确的形态动力学标志物来区分胚胎质量。

第 3 章进一步研究和验证了时差成像技术有助于选择"顶级"胚胎进行移植，以改善 ART 结局，而不是传统的形态学评估。一些用时差成像技术的新研究，评估了胚胎的性别、胚胎碎片化、处理方案、不同的培养基与胚胎形态动力学之间可能存在的相关性；此外，还讨论了在 ART 周期中用时差成像技术设计的各种算法和预测模型。例如，通过普通形态学观察，对动物和人类胚胎发育速度的大量研究表明，男性胚胎比女性胚胎生长得更快[25-27]。虽然女性胚胎表现出晚期分裂（t8）、桑葚胚（tM）和囊胚期的形态动力学参数，但它们呈现出比男性胚胎更早的扩张。不论如何，目前的时差成像技术可能会提供更多关于男性胚胎和女性胚胎在早期分裂过程中的细节差异和确切信息。因此，观察的关键时间点与胚胎性别发育相关。有趣的是，有研究者根据第二次同步时间和桑葚胚形成的时间，设计了一个有 4 个亚组的模型来预测胚胎为雌性的概率。

为了进一步研究和探索胚胎分裂的形态动力学，第 4 章讨论了体外胚胎分裂的一些时空分析方法。在胚胎分裂阶段对早期胚胎图像进行自动或半自动的时差成像分析，可以深入了解有丝分裂时间、卵裂时间和模式等规律。同时，监测分子过程使研究基因表达与细胞生理和发育之间的联系成为可能。通过时差成像数据和分析软件，可以很容易地创建一个四维视频排序的胚胎，从而提供胚胎生长发育过程中时间依赖性的新见解。第 4 章还描述了三种在硬件和软件分析方面不同的方法。对这三种不同的硬件和软件分析方法进行了描述，并举出了一些有结果的例子作为胚胎分裂模式和系谱的体内研究，为胚胎发育学研究打开了一个新窗口。

1.2　通过培养基分析对卵裂期胚胎的基因表达及发育潜能进行无创评估

植入前胚胎发育经历了一系列的关键事件和显著的表观遗传学修饰，基因表达的重编程激活了配子基因组。在植入前胚胎发育的早期阶段，母源 mRNAs 指导胚胎发育。在整个早期胚胎发育过程中，保持着不同的甲基化模式，尽管有些甲基化模式表现出阶段性的变化。最近的研究表明，不同的去甲基化过程导致早期发育胚胎中亲本基因表达的差异，这可能对正常的发育产生影响[28]。另外，非编码 RNAs、长链非编码 RNAs（lncRNA）和短链非编码 RNAs、miRNA 已被证明在 mRNAs 的调控中发挥了重要作用，它们在着床前胚胎发育中具有重要意义。第 5 章综述了着床前胚胎发育过程中影响基因表达的不同因素，包括表观遗传因素，重点是配子和植入前胚胎的甲基化谱；另外还对非编码 RNAs 对基因表达的影响进行了全面评估。

由于基因表达在体外培养的胚胎发育过程中出现，植入前胚胎往往需要营养丰富的培养基。胚胎在生长发育过程中需要从培养基中吸收一些重要的营养成分，并通过代谢产生一些副产物作为基因表达的结果。从这个角度来看，胚胎的体外培养也为通过检测残余胚胎培养基中的生物标志物进行无创胚胎评价提供了非常重要的材料。目前开发的

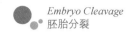

方法集中在测量发育胚胎所分泌的代谢物。这些研究主要利用现代分析学和蛋白质组学的工具。一些研究表明，利用光谱和非光谱对培养基进行代谢分析，可能为目前的胚胎评估策略提供有用的帮助，并对具有发育潜能胚胎表型的观察提供依据[29]。

第 6 章介绍了作为胚胎发育潜能的定量生物标志物人类结合珠蛋白分子的 α-1 链。在一系列回顾性实验中，盲法实验成功率超过 50%。该章总结了目前可用的作为胚胎活力的无创分子评估指标的代谢组学和蛋白质组学方法。最近的研究表明，评估营养介质的分子成分是一个很有前景的领域，可以通过寻找成功植入胚胎、随后的临床妊娠发展和健康婴儿出生的标志以提高使用 ART 技术治疗的效率[30]。如果培养基的分子成分可以作为一个附加的无创移植胚胎选择的标记对胚胎进行选择性移植，它将对改善人类 IVF 的妊娠结果非常有用。

2　改善胚胎分裂的体外培养环境

胚胎质量、分裂速度和基因表达与体外培养环境，包括培养基、培养箱类型和气体浓度，有密切关系[31-32]。因此，自进行胚胎体外培养以来，许多研究都集中在改善胚胎培养条件上。几十年来，优化人类和动物胚胎的培养基一直是人们关注的焦点[33]。目前，有许多商业化的培养基用于人类胚胎培养，它们对胚胎培养的影响各不相同。比较这些培养基对胚胎发育影响的研究报告了相互矛盾的结论，许多研究没有发现这些培养基对胚胎发育的影响有明显的差异，或者只是发现各种培养基之间存在微小的差异[34]。最近，Mantikou 等[35]使用荟萃分析对 20 种不同的培养基进行了 31 项不同的比较，但无法找到哪种培养基具有 IVF/ICSI 的最佳成功率。

此外，IVF 实验室的培养箱在提供稳定和适当的培养环境方面起着关键的作用，这是优化胚胎发育和临床结果所必需的。随着技术的进步，多种类型的培养箱已被应用于人类 IVF 实验室。最近，Swain[32]对人类 IVF 实验室中的胚胎培养箱进行了比较分析，并回顾了一些培养箱的功能和关键环境变量的控制以及各种设备所使用的技术。这一比较表明，较小的台式/顶置式培养箱能提供更快的环境变量恢复，但根据临床结果，任何特定的培养箱都没有明显的优势。

然而，根据过去 10 年的 IVF 临床实践观察，武彬博士的实验室发现了一个有趣的现象，即个别患者的胚胎对培养基和培养箱有特殊的选择响应。部分患者的胚胎在一种培养基中生长良好，但在另一种培养基中却不尽如人意。本书第 7 章对该研究结果做了详细报告。因此，在人类 IVF 临床实践中，使用两种培养基和两种培养箱进行胚胎培养，可以显著提高 IVF/ICSI 的胚胎质量，提高妊娠率。

参考文献

[1] FRAGOULI E, ALFARAWATI S, SPATH K, et al. Morphological and cytogenetic

assessment of cleavage and blastocyst stage embryos [J]. Molecular human reproduction, 2014, 20 (92): 117-126.

[2] KIRKEGAARD K, AHLSTRON A, INGERSLEY H J, et al. Choosing the best embryo by time lapse versus standard morphology [J]. Fertility and sterility, 2015, 103 (2): 323-332.

[3] STRNAD P, GUNTHER S, REICHMANN J, et al. Inverted light-sheet microscope for imaging mouse pre-implantation development [J]. Nature methods, 2016, 13 (2): 139-142.

[4] CHHETRI R K, AMAT F, WAN Y, et al. Whole-animal functional and developmental imaging with isotropic spatial resolution [J]. Nature methods, 2015, 12 (12): 1171-1178.

[5] BRACHETM A. Recherches sur la déterminisme héreditaire de l'oeuf des mammifères. Développement in vitro de jeunes vésicules blastodermiques de lapin [J]. Archives de biologie (Liège), 1913 (28): 423-426.

[6] BIGGERS J D. IVF and embryo transfer: historical origin and development [J]. Fertility magazine, 2012, 25 (5): 118-127.

[7] WHITTEN W K. Culture of tubal mouse ova [J]. Nature, 1956, 177 (4498): 96.

[8] LUNDIN K, BERGH C, HARDARSON T. Early embryo cleavage is a strong indicator of embryo quality in human IVF [J]. Human reproduction, 2001, 16 (2): 2652-2657.

[9] PAYNE J F, RABURN D J, COUCHMAN G M, et al. Relationship between pre-embryo pronuclear morphology (zygote score) and standard day 2 or 3 embryo morphology with regard to assisted reproductive technique outcomes [J]. Fertility and sterility, 2005, 84 (4): 900-909.

[10] ROCOWSKY C, VERNON M, MAYER J, et al. Standardization of grading embryo morphology [J]. Journal of assisted reproduction and genetics, 2010, 27 (8): 437-439.

[11] WU B, TONG J, LEIBO S P. Effect of cooling germinal vesicle-stage bovine oocytes on meiotic spindle formation following in vitro maturation [J]. Molecular reproduction and development, 1999, 54 (4): 388-395.

[12] WU B. Expression of c-fos and c-jun proto-oncogenes by ovine preimplantation embryos [J]. Zygote, 1993, 4 (3): 211-217.

[13] WU B, IGNOTZ G, CURRIE W B, et al. Dynamics of maturation-promoting factor and its constituent proteins during in vitro maturation of bovine oocytes [J]. Biology of reproduction. 1997, 56 (1): 253-259.

[14] WU B, IGNOTZ G, CURRIE W B, et al. Expression of Mos proto-oncoprotein in bovine oocytes during maturation in vitro [J]. Biology of reproduction, 1997, 56 (1): 260-265.

[15] PUISSANT F, RYSSELBERG M V, BARLOW P, et al. Embryo scoring as a prognostic tool in IVF treatment [J]. Human reproduction, 1987, 2 (8): 705-708.

[16] FILHO S E, NOBLE J A, WELLS D. A review on automatic analysis of human embryo

microscope image [J]. The open biomedical engineering journal, 2010, 4: 170-177.

[17] MOLINA I, LÁZARO-IBÁÑEZ E, PERTUSA J, et al. A minimally invasive methodology based on morphometric parameters for day 2 embryo quality assessment [J]. Reproductive biomedicine online, 2014, 29 (4): 470-480.

[18] BRAGA D P A F, SETTI A S, FIGUERIA R C S, et al. The importance of the cleavage stage morphology evaluation for blastocyst transfer in patients with good prognosis [J]. Journal of assisted reproduction and genetics, 2014, 31 (8): 1105-1110.

[19] SALLAM H N, SALLAM N H, SALLAM S H. Non-invasive methods for embryo selection [J]. Facts, views & vision in ObGyn, 2016, 8 (2): 87-100.

[20] UDAN R S, PIAZZA V G, HSU C W, et al. Quantitative imaging of cell dynamics in mouse embryos using light-sheet microscopy [J]. Development, 2014, 141 (22): 4406-4414.

[21] RUBIO I, KUHLMANN R, AGERHOLM I, et al. Limited implantation success of direct-cleaved human zygotes: a time-lapse study [J]. Fertility and sterility, 2012, 98 (6): 1458-1463.

[22] MESEGUER M, RUBIO I, CRUZ M, et al. Embryo incubation and selection in a time-lapse monitoring system improves pregnancy outcome compared with a standard incubator: a retrospective cohort study [J]. Fertility and sterility, 2012, 98 (6): 1481-1489.

[23] DOMINGUEZ F, MESEGUER M, APARICIO-RUIZ B, et al. New strategy for diagnosing embryo implantation potential by combining proteomics and time-lapse technologies [J]. Fertility and sterility, 2015, 104 (4): 908-914.

[24] ZHAN Q S, YE Z, CLARKE R, et al. Direct unequal cleavages: embryo developmental competence, genetic constitution and clinical outcome [J]. Plos one, 2016, 11 (12): e0166398.

[25] WU B. Amplification of the Sry gene allows identification of the sex of mouse preimplantation embryos [J]. Theriogenology, 1993, 40: 441-453.

[26] ALFARAWATI S, FRAGOULI E, COLLS P, et al. The relationship between blastocyst morphology, chromosomal abnormality, and embryo gender [J]. Fertility and sterility, 2011, 95 (2): 520-524.

[27] HENTEMANN M A, BRISKEMYR S, BERTHEUSSEN K. Blastocyst transfer and gender: IVF versus ICSI [J]. Journal of assisted reproduction and genetics, 2009, 26 (8): 433-436.

[28] OSWALD J, ENGEMANN S, LANE N, et al. Active demethylation of the paternal genome in the mouse zygote [J]. Current biology: CB, 2000, 10 (8): 475-478.

[29] BOTROS L, SAKKAS D, SELI E. Metabolomics and its application for non-invasive embryo assessment in IVF [J]. Molecular human reproduction, 2008, 14 (12): 679-690.

[30] ZORINA Z I M, SMOLNIKOVA S V Y, BOBROV B M Y. Study of embryo metabolic products in culture media as a tool for determining the implantation potential [J]. Akusherstvo i Ginekologiia, 2017, 2: 11 – 16.

[31] LONERGAN P, RIZOS D, GUTIÉRREZ-ADÁN A, et al. Effect of culture environment on embryo quality and gene expression: experience from animal studies [J]. Reproductive biomedicine online, 2003, 7 (6): 657 – 663.

[32] SWAIN J E. Optimal human embryo culture [J]. Seminars in reproductive medicine, 2015, 33 (2): 103 – 117.

[33] BIGGERS J D. Thoughts on embryo culture conditions [J]. Reproductive biomedicine online, 2002, 4 (Suppl 1): 30 – 38.

[34] AOKI V W, WILCOX A L, PETERSON C M, et al. Comparison of four media types during 3-day human IVF embryo culture [J]. Reproductive biomedicine online, 2005, 10 (5): 600 – 606.

[35] MANTIKOU E, YOUSSEF M A F M, VAN WELY M, et al. Embryo culture media and IVF/ICSI success rates: a systematic review [J]. Human reproduction update, 2013, 19 (3): 210 – 220.

(Bin Wu)

第 2 章 胚胎分裂时间轴

> 时差成像可以提供一个连续观察胚胎发育的培养环境。有许多形态动力学标记可以帮助我们找出最佳质量的胚胎。我们回顾了相关研究，用以阐明胚胎着床潜能与胚胎染色体状态之间的标记关系。令人惊讶的是，大多数标记对着床潜能和妊娠率的影响是有争议的，或没有显著影响。我们认为一些不确定的因素可能影响胚胎着床和妊娠。在此，我们提供了一种新的胚胎优选方法，该方法通过时差成像中的许多形态动力学标记来选择最佳质量的胚胎。因此，我们可以预期，时差成像可以帮助我们选择优质的胚胎进行后续移植，以提高着床潜能、染色体整倍性和妊娠率。此外，还需要对母体条件与胚胎着床的相关性进行研究。

胚胎形态观察是辅助生殖技术（ART）中选择高着床潜能胚胎的最广泛的方法。传统上，在受精后每天观察胚胎发育情况，可以帮助胚胎学家选择最佳质量的胚胎进行移植，最终提高活产率。然而，由于形态学观察需要将胚胎在培养箱与外部环境之间频繁转移，日常观察被认为对胚胎发育不利。因此，一种新的技术——时差成像（TLI），被开发用以预测胚胎的形态动力学标记。目前，时差成像可用于评估从受精到囊胚的胚胎生长状态。通过每 5～20 min 自动获取一次图像，针对原核、卵裂期和囊胚形态进行连续的形态学评估。此外，由于绕过了日常观察，时差成像提供了一个稳定的培养条件。本章将讨论胚胎分裂的时间对着床潜能的影响。

1 形态学标记

一般来说，从受精到囊胚形成期间有许多里程碑事件发生，包括原核出现、原核消失、受精卵第一次分裂、受精卵第二次分裂和囊胚形成（图 2-1）。由于拍摄时间限制，时差成像无法获得每一分钟的照片。虽然时差成像的局限性是显而易见的，但目前它仍然是评估胚胎发育时间的最实用方式。下面列举了形态动力学标记，并讨论了胚胎发育过程中不同时间节点对临床结局的影响。

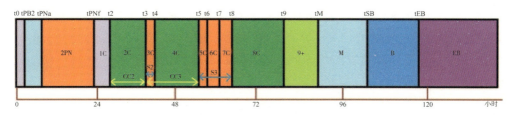

tPB2：第二极体排出的时间；tPNa：原核出现的时间；tPNf：原核消失的时间；t2、t3、t4、t5、t6、t7、t8、t9：从受精到二、三、四、五、六、七、八、九细胞期的时间；tM：从受精到桑葚胚的时间；tSB：从受精到囊胚形成的时间；tEB：从受精到扩张囊胚的时间；cc2：t3 - t2；cc3：t5 - t3；s3：t8 - t5。

图 2 - 1　胚胎发育的里程碑事件

(1) 第二极体排出的时间 (tPB2)。ICSI 后 (2.9 ± 0.1) h 是第二极体排出的时间。排出时间范围为 0.7～10.15 h。如果卵母细胞来自大于 38 岁的女性，第二极体排出的时间明显延迟，但在进一步的胚胎发育中没有观察到其他影响[1]。tPB2 的平均时间在整倍体和非整倍体胚胎中分别为 3.9 h 和 4.0 h。胚胎染色体完整性与第二极体排出的时间无关[2]。

(2) 原核出现的时间 (tPNa)。着床组的原核 (pronucleus, PN) 出现时间为 (8.4 ± 2.4) h，未着床组的为 (8.2 ± 1.9) h[3]。在整倍体胚胎和非整倍体胚胎中，tPNa 的平均时间分别为 10.1 h 和 10.2 h。因此，原核出现的时间对着床潜能和染色体整倍性没有明显影响。

(3) 原核消失的时间 (tPNf)。原核消失的时间较长，可能有利于活产。Azzarello 等[4]称，活产组的 tPNf 较没活产的 tPNf 长 [(24.9 ± 0.6) h vs (23.3 ± 0.4) h]，当 PN 消失的时间少于 20 h，则没有活产。着床组胚胎和未着床组胚胎的原核消失时间相等[3,5]。tPNf 在整倍体胚胎中的平均时间为 24.4 h，在非整倍体胚胎中的为 24.8 h[2]。当 tPNf 小于 20 h，原核消失时间对胚胎着床和染色体整倍性无显著差异，但无活产。

(4) 从受精到二细胞期的时间 (t2)。在这个阶段时长对胚胎结局的影响仍存在争议。Meseguer 等[6]提出，着床组胚胎的 t2 比未着床组胚胎的 t2 小 [(25.6 ± 2.2) h vs (26.7 ± 3.8) h]。Chamayou 等[3]研究显示，着床组胚胎的 t2 和未着床组胚胎的 t2 没有明显差异 [(26.9 ± 3.2) h vs (27.0 ± 4.0) h]。Kirkegaard 等[5]发现，妊娠组的 t2 和非妊娠组的 t2 是类似的。奇怪的是，胚胎在单一培养基中培养时的 t2 比在序贯培养基中培养时的 t2 小 [(27.36 ± 4.12) h vs (29.09 ± 4.86) h][7]。t2 在整倍体胚胎和非整倍体胚胎中 (28 h vs 28.4 h) 没有显著差异[2]。在着床组胚胎中，达到二细胞期的耗时可能更短，但在染色体整倍性方面没有显著性。

(5) 从受精到三细胞、四细胞、五细胞期的时间 (t3、t4、t5)。一些研究表明，在较短的 t3、t4 和 t5 中观察到胚胎着床潜能的增强。着床组胚胎的 t3、t4 和 t5 明显小于未着床组胚胎的。着床组胚胎的 t3 [(37.4 ± 2.8) h]、t4 [(38.2 ± 3.0) h] 和 t5 [(52.3 ± 4.2) h] 与未着床组胚胎的 t3 [(38.4 ± 5.2) h]、t4 [(40.0 ± 5.4) h] 和 t5 [(52.6 ± 6.8) h] 相比有显著性差异[6]。然而，Chamayou[3] 和 Kirkegaard 等[5]证明在胚胎着床和妊娠率方面，t3、t4 和 t5 没有差异。在单一培养基中培养的胚胎比在序贯培养基中培养的胚胎发育更快 [t3,(37.75 ± 6.64) h vs (39.53 ± 6.15) h;t4,(40.07 ± 5.98) h

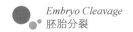

vs（41.45±6.07）h；t5,（48.77±9.49）h vs（52.22±9.34）h][7]。整倍体胚胎和非整倍体胚胎的 t3（37.4 h vs 37.2 h）和 t5（50.4 h vs 50.6 h）没有显著性差异，但 t4 在整倍体胚胎和非整倍体胚胎中（40.0 h vs 41.1 h）有显著性差异[2]。因此，t3、t4、t5 的胚胎发育较快，有利于着床，但只有 t4 可能影响囊胚的整倍体率。

（6）从受精到六细胞、七细胞、八细胞、九细胞期的时间（t6、t7、t8、t9）。根据以往的报道，虽然 t8 在着床组胚胎中表现得更快［(54.9±5.2) h vs (58.0±7.2) h][8]，但另一份报告显示，着床组胚胎和未着床组胚胎在 t6 ［(54.3±5.8) h vs (54.5±8.2) h］、t7 ［(57.4±8.6) h vs (57.6±9.8) h］、t8 ［(61.0±10.8) h vs (60.8±11.5) h］ 和 t9 ［(77.0±8.5) h vs (76.0±11.3) h] 之间的差异没有统计学意义[3]。此外，Kirkegaard 等[5]也证明妊娠率与这一时期无关。整倍体胚胎的 t6（53.9 h）、t7（57.8 h）、t8（61.9 h）和 t9（76.1 h）与非整倍体胚胎相似[2]。从统计学上看，t6、t7、t8 和 t9 在着床组胚胎和未着床组胚胎以及在整倍体胚胎和非整倍体胚胎之间没有显著性差异。

（7）从受精到桑葚胚的时间（tM）。桑葚胚是指所有细胞融合在一起的胚胎。着床组胚胎和未着床组胚胎的 tM 分别为（86.0±9.1）h 和（84.4±11.4）h，没有统计学差异[3]。整倍体（94.4 h）和非整倍体（95.3 h）胚胎的 tM 也无显著性差异[2]。因此，在统计学上，tM 并不影响着床潜能和染色体整倍性。

（8）从受精到囊胚形成的时间（tSB）。囊胚形成指的是观察到囊胚腔的时间点。着床和妊娠的平均 tSB 没有明显差异[3,5]。因此，从受精到囊胚形成的时间并不影响胚胎的着床潜能和妊娠率。然而，整倍体胚胎的平均 tSB（103.4 h）明显短于非整倍体胚胎的 tSB（105.0 h，$P=0.007$）[2]。此外，较短的 tSB 关系到选择整倍体胚胎进行胚胎移植的机会更大。

（9）从受精到扩张囊胚的时间（tEB）。扩张囊胚是指囊胚的直径增加了 30% 以上，扩张的结果是透明带变薄[9]。着床组胚胎的 tEB 和未着床组胚胎的 tEB 没有统计学差异（111.7 h vs 110.5 h）[3]。Kirkegaard 等[5]也指出，妊娠组和非妊娠组的 tEB 没有显著性差异。然而，整倍体胚胎的平均 tEB 明显小于非整倍体胚胎（118.7 h vs 122.1 h）[2]。此外，囊胚扩张用时较短的胚胎更有可能是整倍体胚胎，但在 tEB、着床潜能和妊娠方面没有差异。

（10）二细胞期和三细胞期之间的时间（t3-t2，cc2）。二细胞期和三细胞期之间的时间段也被称为分裂周期二。着床组胚胎 cc2 的平均值为 11.4 h，未着床组胚胎 cc2 的平均值为 11.8 h[3]。Meseguer 等[6]发现着床组胚胎 cc2 和未着床组胚胎 cc2 相同（11.8 h）。平均 cc2（11.0 h）在妊娠组和未妊娠组之间也没有显著性差异[5]。整倍体胚胎和非整倍体胚胎的平均 cc2 也没有显著性差异（10.5 h vs 10.4 h）[2]。因此，cc2 不能预测着床潜能、妊娠率和染色体整倍性。

（11）三细胞期和五细胞期之间的时间（t3-t5，cc3）。Chamayou 等[3]也将其定义为分裂周期三。他们提出，着床组胚胎 cc3 的中位数明显长于未着床组胚胎的 cc3（14.4 h vs 13.0 h）。因此，较长的 cc3 可能有利于胚胎的发育。

（12）第二个细胞周期的同步时间段（s2，t4-t3）。三细胞期和四细胞期之间的时间段即 s2。着床组胚胎的 s2 平均值为 2.0 h，未着床组胚胎的 s2 平均值为 1.7 h[3]。s2 平均值在妊娠组和非妊娠组之间也没有显著性差异[5]。然而，整倍体胚胎的 s2 平均值明显小于非整倍体胚胎的 s2 平均值（2.6 h vs 4.2 h）[2]。因此，s2 的平均值可用于预测胚胎的染色体整倍性。

（13）第三个细胞周期的同步时间段（s3，t8 - t5）。s3 是五细胞期和八细胞期之间的时间段。它包括五细胞、六细胞和七细胞期的时间总和。着床组胚胎的平均 s3 和未着床组胚胎的平均 s3 没有显著性差异（8.0 h vs 8.1 h）[3]。Kirkegaard 等[5] 也发现妊娠组的 s3 和非妊娠组的 s3 没有显著性差异。没有数据对整倍体胚胎 s3 和非整倍体胚胎 s3 的平均值进行比较。因此，s3 对着床潜能和妊娠率的影响不显著。

2 时差成像中的特殊标记

通过连续和频繁的记录，一些形态动力学标记在时差成像中显示出来。传统的观察方法很难观察到这些短暂的现象。下面列出了这些形态动力学标记，并总结了其对胚胎的影响。

（1）直接分裂（从二细胞期的时间到三细胞期的时间 ≤5 h）：一般来说，从二细胞期到三细胞期的时间为 10～11 h[2-3,5-6]。Rubio 等[10] 发现，直接分裂（≤5 h）的胚胎比正常分裂模式的胚胎种植率低（1.2% vs 20.0%）。直接分裂的发生率为 14%。导致直接分裂的原因仍不清楚。根据 Rubio 等[10] 的报道，由精子引入的中心粒控制着卵母细胞的第一次有丝分裂。因此，在 ICSI 过程中，精子颈部的损伤，即中心粒的位置受损，可能会改变胚胎第一次分裂的时间。不选择直接分裂的胚胎进行移植可以提高种植率。

（2）直接不均匀分裂（direct unequal cleavage，DUC）：实际上，直接不均匀分裂可能发生在任何分裂周期。Zhan 等[11] 将其定义为一个胚胎突然分裂为 3 个子胚胎或细胞周期的间隔小于 5 h。因此，将第一次分裂时的直接不均匀分裂描述为 DUC1，在第二次分裂时描述为 DUC2，在第三次分裂时描述为 DUC3，将显示多个 DUC 的胚胎描述为 DUC Plus。他们发现，用附睾和睾丸的精子受精的胚胎具有明显较高的 DUC1 发生率（13.6% vs 11.4%）。然而，在用射精的精子受精的胚胎中，DUC1 的发生率为 9.1%。此外，胚胎分裂球多核（multinucleation blastomere，MNB）的发生率是非 MNB 的 2～3 倍。他们的结论是，DUC 胚胎的囊胚率、着床潜能和整倍体率都显著降低。非 DUC 胚胎应作为胚胎移植的首选。

（3）反向分裂：反向分裂可分为两种类型。反向分裂类型 1（完全）：卵裂球完全分离后重新结合。反向分裂类型 2（不完全）：受精卵或卵裂球未能分离（类型 1，补充视频 1；类型 2，补充视频 2；可于 www.fertstert.org 在线获得）。在前 3 个分裂周期中，27.4% 的胚胎可能发生多达 3 次的反向分裂[12]。与促性腺激素释放激素（gonadotropin-releasing hormone，GnRH）激动剂方案和 IVF 受精相比，GnRH 拮抗剂方案和 ICSI 受精有更高的反向分裂发生率。精子活力差（<21%）的受精胚胎也有较高的反向分裂发生率。此外，有反向分裂的胚胎与分级较差胚胎和较低的着床潜能有关。因此，反向卵裂是胚胎选择的一个负面因素。

3　结论

胚胎发育的持续形态动力学变化是时差成像的主要特征。我们可以观察到胚胎发育的许多关键节点，并计算出时间间隔，以了解其和着床潜能、染色体整倍性以及妊娠率的关系。遗憾的是，所有的形态动力学标记都不能准确预测着床潜能、染色体整倍性和妊娠率。大多数标记是有争议的或没有显著的影响。一般来说，建议选择发育较快的胚胎进行移植以提高妊娠率。但是，数据显示并不是所有的标记都能支持这一原则。

对标记的描述存在争议的原因是多方面的。有些因素可能会影响胚胎的着床和妊娠。母体的身体状态，如子宫内膜容受性、子宫内膜息肉、子宫内膜或宫颈感染、水肿、免疫紊乱、亚临床甲状腺功能减退等，也会阻碍胚胎着床和随后的妊娠。非整倍体胚胎的种植率很低或会导致自然流产。虽然一些标记与较高的整倍体胚胎率相关，但它仍然不能准确预测整倍体胚胎。如果胚胎学家想知道胚胎的染色体状况，植入前遗传学筛查（PGS）仍然是首选。

因此，时差成像可以帮助我们评估胚胎的质量，使用更精确的形态动力学标记来评价胚胎的质量。质量好的胚胎有更高的着床潜能和正常的染色体。目前，PGS 是发现整倍体胚胎的最佳方式。然而，高质量的整倍体胚胎并不能保证着床和妊娠，而只是胚胎着床的基本条件。必须考虑许多其他的母体生理情况，以提高种植率和妊娠率，这也需要进一步的研究来阐明着床过程的奥秘。

参考文献

[1] LIU Y H, CHAPPLE V, ROBERTS P, et al. Time-lapse videography of human oocytes following intracytoplasmic sperm injection: events up to the first cleavage division [J]. Reproductive biology, 2014, 14 (4): 249 – 256.

[2] MINASI M G, COLASANTE A, RICCIO T, et al. Correlation between aneuploidy, standard morphology evaluation and morphokinetic development in 1730 biopsied blastocysts: a consecutive case series study [J]. Human reproduction, 2016, 31 (10): 2245 – 2254.

[3] CHAMAYOU S, PATRIZIO P, STORACI G, et al. The use of morphokinetic parameters to select all embryos with full capacity to implant [J]. Journal of assisted reproduction and genetics, 2013, 30 (5): 703 – 710.

［4］AZZARELLO A, HOEST T, MIKKELSEN A L. The impact of pronuclei morphology and dynamicity on live birth outcome after time-lapse culture［J］. Human reproduction, 2012, 27（9）: 2649-2657.

［5］KIRKEGAARD K, KESMODEL U S, HINDKJAER J J, et al. Time-lapse parameters as predictors of blastocyst development and pregnancy outcome in embryos from good prognosis patients: a prospective cohort study［J］. Human reproduction, 2013, 28（10）: 2643-2651.

［6］MESEGUER M, HERRERO J, TEJERA A, et al. The use of morphokinetic as a predictor of embryo implantation［J］. Human reproduction, 2011, 26（10）: 2658-2671.

［7］CIRAY H N, AKSOY T, GOKTAS C, et al. Time-lapse evaluation of human embryo development in single versus sequential culture media—a sibling oocyte study［J］. Journal of assisted reproduction and genetics, 2012, 29（9）: 891-900.

［8］DAL CANTO M, COTICCHIO G, RENZINI M M, et al. Cleavage kinetics analysis of human embryos predicts development to blastocyst and implantation［J］. Reproductive biomedicine online, 2012, 25（5）: 474-480.

［9］CAMPBELL A, FISHEL S, BOWMAN N, et al. Modelling a risk classification of aneuploidy in human embryos using non-invasive morphokinetics［J］. Reproductive biomedicine online, 2013, 26（5）: 477-485.

［10］RUBIO I, KUHLMANN R, AGERHOLM I, et al. Limited implantation success of direct-cleaved human zygotes: a time-lapse study［J］. Fertility and sterility, 2012, 98（6）: 1458-1463.

［11］ZHAN Q S, YE Z, CLARKE R, et al. Direct unequal cleavages: Embryo developmental competence, genetic constitution and clinical outcome［J］. Plos one, 2016, 11（12）: e0166398.

［12］LIU Y H, CHAPPLE V, ROBERTS P, et al. Prevalence, consequence, and significance of reverse cleavage by human embryos viewed with the use of the Embryoscope time-lapse video system［J］. Fertility and sterility, 2014, 102（5）: 1295-1300.

（Meng Ju Lee）

第3章 基于时差成像观测的胚胎形态动力学研究

> 胚胎培养和评估是辅助生殖技术的关键步骤。通常,胚胎学家在胚胎培养期间需要从传统培养箱中移出胚胎在显微镜下进行胚胎评估。近年来出现的时差成像技术可以在胚胎发育的关键点间歇性拍摄胚胎的数字图像。这种技术让胚胎学家可以在稳定的培养环境中评估胚胎质量。根据时差成像研究和事先的算法模型,单独的时差成像或其与常规形态学相结合评估似乎可以用于挑选高质量胚胎,是改善胚胎着床和妊娠率的有效诊断工具。此外,胚胎发育时间点与胚胎性别、胚胎碎片以及卵巢刺激方案类型之间存在显著差异。总之,应对时差成像采取更进一步的研究评估,并应在各个实验室评估其性价比。

辅助生殖技术(ART)可以帮助不育夫妇实现孕育孩子的梦想,但体外受精(IVF)的妊娠率和活产率仍然较低。我们想通过识别具有最高着床潜能的可用胚胎以提高 IVF 成功率。在传统的 IVF 实践中,胚胎评估主要基于胚胎学家对卵母细胞及胚胎发育的各个阶段的形态学观察。卵母细胞、胚胎质量、卵裂球数量和均等性、碎片率、细胞质粒度等一些特征已被定义为预测妊娠成功的指标。这种传统的胚胎评估方法可能会对胚胎生长产生一些不利影响:因为培养箱的频繁开闭往往会引起胚胎培养环境稳定性的变化。IVF 实验室采用时差成像(TLI)技术可以减少观察者之间和观察者自身的差异及变化。时差成像技术在 IVF 实验室的应用为胚胎发育研究提供了更详细的观察资料。

本章的目的是探讨常规形态学评估以外的时差成像,探讨其是否可以选择高质量胚胎进行移植以改善 ART 结局;基于时差成像的一些新研究,可能揭示胚胎性别、胚胎碎片、治疗方案、不同培养基和胚胎形态动力学之间存在的相关性。此外,还将探讨在 ART 周期中时差成像的不同算法和预测模型。

1 时差成像

ART 流程的主要目的是提高移植胚胎的种植率和妊娠率,这一过程受多种因素的影响。其中的一个主要问题是如何在体外培养系统中观察胚胎的生长和发育情况。最近,一种新的具有时差成像功能的胚胎培养系统已经开始用于 IVF 实验室实践中。在这种自动化胚胎学设备中,可以不从培养箱中移出胚胎便可对胚胎发育期间的关键事件进行监测。一方面,时差成像可以在胚胎培养期间保护胚胎免受温度、pH 和湿度等环境变化的影响;另一方面,时差成像可以减少由于胚胎学家的专业知识和能力的差异对胚胎评估产生的误判。通过连续的图像记录,胚胎发育过程中的一些关键事件可以被更完整地记录,并用于胚胎评估。IVF 面临的另一个问题是多胎妊娠,这会增加母亲和胎儿的并发症。在世界范围内,许多 IVF 实验室倾向于选择高发育潜能的胚胎进行移植,通过选择性单胚胎移植(elective single embryo transfer,eSET)来减少移植胚胎的数量。时差成像可以帮助胚胎学家选择最有发育潜能的胚胎,并降低多胎妊娠率。时差成像的应用最初由 Wong 等[1]证明,他们发现胚胎最初的细胞分裂是胚胎评估和胚胎发育预测的工具。接下来,Meseguer 等[2]报道了早期胚胎分裂时间和间隔与胚胎着床能力之间的关系。时差成像是传统胚胎形态学评估的无创替代方法,它利用发育动力学和胚胎形态学,准确观察细胞异常事件,如直接分裂为 3 个细胞、卵裂球融合、多核、碎片重吸收[3]。

1.1 时差形态动力学参数和胚胎着床潜能

1.1.1 支持时差成像预测价值的论据

时差成像结合常规形态学观察胚胎评估可提高种植率和妊娠率。Adamson 等[4]研究了 319 个胚胎移植周期,并将其分为单独标准形态学评估组(对照组)和 TLS 加形态学评估组(实验组)。结果显示,实验组和对照组种植率分别为 30.2% 和 19.0%,临床妊娠率分别为 46.0% 和 32.1%($P<0.05$)。一项历史队列研究表明,在培养的前 48 h 内的 3 种胚胎形态动力学指标(包括第一次胞质分裂、三细胞期的持续时间以及直接分裂为 3 个细胞)与高质量囊胚形成相关[5]。Milewski 等[6]还分析了 1 060 个胚胎的发育数据,认为胚胎形态动力学参数与囊胚形成及胚胎种植率相关,并反映在胚胎质量上。在有生化妊娠、无生化妊娠组和临床妊娠组之间,最大的形态学参数差异是 t9(从受精到第 9 次分裂的时间)、t8_int(第 3 次分裂后的阶段)和 cc4(第 4 次分裂)的平均值的不同。在一项随机、双盲、对照试验中,930 例患者随机分为 2 组,实验组时差成像 2 638 个胚胎与在标准培养箱中培养的对照组 2 427 个胚胎相比,时差成像胚胎的种植率(44.9% 和 37.1%)和持续妊娠率(51.4% 和 41.7%)均显著高于对照组。据报道,与标准培养胚胎相比,在时差成像的胚胎中早期妊娠丢失减少(25.8% 和 16.6%),有

统计学意义[7]。来源于60名患者的648个胚胎，在时差成像培养过程中进行了前瞻性评估。将胚胎培养至第5天（囊胚期），与形成囊胚的胚胎相比，废弃胚胎的早期卵裂分裂时间（t2，t4和t8）、桑葚胚分裂时间（tMor）、囊胚开始形成时间（tSB）、囊胚形成时间（tBL）和扩张囊胚时间（tEBL）显著更长。此外，早期胚胎动力学参数与着床潜能相关，但在晚期胚胎动力学参数中未观察到这种相关性[8]。此外，在一项前瞻性多中心队列研究中，使用时差成像结合早期胚胎活力评估（early embro viability assessment，Eeva），评估了5个IVF中心的1 727个胚胎，主要比较了胚胎学家以Day-3形态学评估与同时应用形态学结合Eeva选择胚胎的差异。3名使用形态学或形态学加Eeva的胚胎学家报道的特异性分别为59.7% vs 86.3%、41.9% vs 84.0%和79.5% vs 86.6%。结果显示，将Eeva与Day-3形态学相结合显著提升了经验丰富的胚胎学家的胚胎识别能力，这些评估手段的有效性甚至可延伸至囊胚期[9]。与此一致的是，另一项研究使用了上述方法，5位胚胎学家也发现了类似的结果。仅使用形态学评估的优势比为1.68（95% CI = 1.29～2.19），而常规形态学与Eeva相结合导致预测囊胚形成的优势比更高，达到2.57（95% CI = 1.88～3.51）。因此，将Eeva添加到传统的胚胎评估中可降低胚胎学家之间的不一致性[10]。此外，在一项大型队列研究中，在TLS培养箱中培养通过ICSI受精的9 530个胚胎。胚胎分组分为常规分裂组、可用八细胞期组、可用囊胚组和植入胚胎组4个亚组进行评估。在t2、t3、t5、cc2、cc3、s2和s3指标上，常规分裂组和可用八细胞期组之间存在显著性差异。t5、t8、tM、cc3和s2的时长在可用囊胚组中显著高于可用八细胞期组。植入胚胎组的t8、tM、tB和s2大于可用囊胚组。结果证实，时差成像在检测胚胎发育和着床潜能方面具有准确性[11]。同样，在一个大样本量的观察性研究中，在时差成像中培养了7 483个经ICSI受精的受精卵。对17种形态动力学参数进行了评估，发现它们与囊胚形成和植入之间存在许多显著的相关性。囊胚形成的最大预后参数包括桑葚胚形成时间（tM）和t8 - t5。这些参数对着床潜能的预测性较差。具有着床潜能预测能力的参数是囊胚扩张的时间（tEB）和t8 - t5 [12]。

1.1.2 反对时差成像预测价值的论点

在一项随机对照试验中，Park等[13]对封闭式时差成像中240例患者与常规培养箱中的124例患者进行比较，认为四细胞期的胚胎数量、种植率和持续妊娠率没有显著性差异，并发现时差成像组的流产率明显较高。这些结果与其他研究的结果一致，这些研究显示，常规培养组与时差成像组之间在优胚率、胚胎发育速度、成囊率、种植率以及持续妊娠率方面没有显著性差异[14-16]。一项由2部分组成的研究显示，预后不良的患者在时差成像系统和传统培养胚胎之间的第3天胚胎质量、种植率和临床妊娠率方面没有差异；而在第二部分，与常规培养的胚胎相比，在时差成像培养箱中的胚胎在发育至第3天时质量明显较差[17]。最近的一项研究报道，通过常规形态学评估或时差成像评估了2 092个接受IVF周期的胚胎，结果显示，移植第5天胚胎的临床妊娠率是移植第3天的胚胎的3倍。但传统组和时差成像组的临床妊娠率（68% vs 63%）和种植率（51% vs 45%）相当[18]。

总之，基于时间和异常形态事件出现的新指标只能通过时差成像来确认。在早期胚胎发育阶段检测到的许多标记可以为胚胎选择提供早期的、有效的判断依据。此外，时差成像观察到的动力学参数似乎可以预测囊胚形成高发育潜能。因此,应该进行更多、更准确的荟萃分析研究,以帮助胚胎学家选择具有高着床潜能的胚胎。

1.2　性别对胚胎形态动力学的影响

有一种假设认为,在男性胚胎和女性胚胎之间胚胎发育阶段是有差异的,在动物研究中也有类似报道[19-20]。据报道,对于人类胚胎,男性胚胎生长速度比女性胚胎快[21-22],但也有研究否定了这一理论[23-24]。目前,用于观察胚胎发育过程的时差成像可以在胚胎早期分裂期间监测胚胎。回顾性观察78例女性胚胎和60例男性胚胎,移植的全部胚胎均使用时差成像培养并鉴定性别状况,结果显示,女性胚胎呈现出比男性胚胎更早扩张的趋势。但其他关键时间点、时间间隔与囊胚形成率大致相同[23]。研究分析了通过ART周期分娩的81名新生儿,结果显示,女性胚胎与晚期卵裂(t8)、桑葚胚形成时间(tM)和囊胚期阶段形态动力学参数有关,部分扩张囊胚阶段的形态动力学参数与胚胎性别(女性)相关[25]。另一项研究中评估了176个男性胚胎和161个女性胚胎,胚胎发育时间点及时间间隔与性别有显著差异,研究根据第二次同步时间和桑葚胚形成时间设计了一个模型,并用4个亚组来预测胚胎是女性的概率[26]。综上,还需要更大样本,进一步研究以确定胚胎形态动力学与性别之间的关系。

1.3　碎片对胚胎形态动力学的影响

胚胎碎片是早期胚胎发育阶段的常见模式。在常规的形态学胚胎评估中,高度碎片化的胚胎由于着床潜能低而不适合移植或冷冻保存[27]。在没有时差成像的情况下,胚胎在培养期间发生的碎片数量和体积的变化无法观察到。近年来,时差成像的应用为获得更多特定时间点的胚胎生长的信息提供了依据。Stensen等[28]分别使用PolScope仪器和时差成像评估了1943个卵母细胞和372个胚胎。研究显示,在受精后42～45 h具有小于10%碎片(低比例碎片)的胚胎与减数分裂纺锤体早期出现、快速第一次有丝分裂、第二次有丝分裂开始较晚和第三次有丝分裂有较小周期的胚胎有关;可是,大于50%碎片(高比例碎片)的胚胎与减数分裂纺锤体出现较晚[注射人绒毛膜促性腺激素(human chorionic gonadotrophin,HCG)36.5 h后]、延迟启动第一次有丝分裂(受精后29.8 h)、第二次有丝分裂的启动较早(受精后36.4 h)和第三次有丝分裂细胞周期的间隔更长的胚胎有关。研究显示,早期胚胎发育阶段的碎片与错误的有丝分裂有关[27]。Stensen的研究认为,在形态学评估中,高度碎片化的胚胎,在第一次有丝分裂时碎片不能被重新吸收。根据上述数据,在体外培养中,胚胎的碎片与减数分裂和有丝分裂过程之间存在相关性。

1.4　卵巢刺激方案对胚胎形态动力学的影响

卵母细胞和胚胎的质量在体外培养周期中受多种因素的影响,其中一个重要因素是在ART周期中的卵巢刺激治疗方案,另外也受患者的生理状况和临床医生决定的影响。用于卵巢刺激的促性腺激素,增加了卵泡液中的激素水平和卵丘细胞的凋亡[29]。近年来,在卵巢刺激方案中,使用时差成像评估不同药物和剂量对胚胎质量的影响。

Munoz[30] 等回顾性分析了使用时差成像观察捐卵周期中的 2 817 个胚胎，发现由 GnRH 拮抗剂 + GnRH 激动剂刺激的周期所产生的胚胎分裂比来自用 GnRH 激动剂 + HCG 治疗的患者的胚胎分裂更快；但是，除了第一个发育阶段外，其他阶段差异并不显著。此外，另一项回顾性研究观察了 739 个胚胎，使用时差成像比较了使用 HCG 和 GnRHa 治疗的患者的胚胎形态动力学差异，发现和 HCG 周期相比，GnRHa 周期胚胎发育更迟缓[31]。与上述研究不同，使用 TLS 分析 3 个研究组［仅使用重组促卵泡激素（recombinant follicle stimulating hormone，rFSH）治疗患者组、仅使用人类绝经期促性腺激素（human menopausal gonadotropin，HMG）组、rFSH 与 HMG 组合使用组］的胚胎形态动力学特征，没有发现显著差异。rFSH 组的时间点和时间间隔均接近理想时间，没有显著性差异[32]。根据上述有限的研究得出的结论是卵巢刺激方案的类型以不同的模式影响胚胎发育动力学。

1.5 培养基类型对胚胎形态动力学的影响

培养基成分和培养条件已被证实对胚胎发育是至关重要的。目前，使用时差成像可以准确地看到培养基对胚胎形态动力学的影响。使用时差成像的动物研究证实，不同成分的培养基对囊胚形成有影响[33]。在一项队列研究中，使用 2 种不同的培养基培养 532 个人类胚胎，Global 为连续培养基，Sage 为序贯培养基。通过时差成像监测受精到二细胞期（t2）、三细胞期（t3）、四细胞期（t4）和五细胞期（t5），同时监测二细胞维持时长（cc2）和三细胞维持时长（s2）。2 种培养基的胚胎在上述时间点无显著差异。种植率和妊娠率在各组之间也无明显差异[34]。对 1 356 个胚胎的随机临床试验结果与上述研究结果相似：将所有受精卵随机分为连续培养基培养和序贯培养基培养 2 组，并在时差成像中监测至第 5 天，第 5 天两组间的优质囊胚的百分比相当。然而，在连续培养基中，第 3 天优质胚胎的数量显著增加。对 11 个形态动力学参数进行评估显示：只有 4 个参数（t7，t8，t3c4c——第一次观察 3～4 个完全分离的卵裂球的时间，t5c7c——第一次观察 5～7 个完全分离的卵裂球的时间）在不同培养基培养的胚胎之间有显著性差异，认为连续培养基和序贯培养基对囊胚发育的影响无统计学差异[35]。Costa-Borges 等[36] 比较在第 3 天更换培养基与不更换培养基的胚胎形态动力学参数。结果显示，两者的优质囊胚率、囊胚形成率、胚胎早期和晚期形态动力学参数，以及临床妊娠率、出生率及围生期结局均没有显著性差异。

根据有限的研究，序贯培养基和连续培养基对胚胎形态动力学方面具有大致同等的效果。当然，需要进一步的研究来支持这一理论。

1.6 用于预测胚胎着床潜能的形态动力学算法

时差成像的发展提供了连续观察胚胎发育的方式，胚胎学家可以使用基于胚胎形态动力学的新评分系统选择质量最好的胚胎，但是目前需要全球公认的算法来预测胚胎着床潜能。Meseguer 等[37] 首先提出早期胚胎形态动力学的分级模型。他们将 247 个胚胎分为 6 个小组，其中 4 个小组进一步细分为 2 个小类，根据胚胎的着床潜能进行分类，设计了多变量模型。4 年后，Freour 等[38] 的一项回顾性研究评估验证了该模型。他们计算了与 Meseguer 模型设计的每个相匹配亚组的种植率，并根据胚胎移植的日期分析了亚组中的相似数据。根据形态动力学亚组，Meseguer 模型对种植率的预测没有显示出同样的灵敏度。为建立时差选择模型，基于定性和定量参数，他们回顾性分析了 270 个已知植入胚胎的数据（known implantation data，KID），随后对 66 枚 KID 进行了评估以验证模型。定性的非选择参数描述为：第 3 天常规形态差，实时观察系统检测到异常卵裂模式，在受精后 68 h 内少于 8 个细胞。定量参数为：从原核消失（pronuclear fading，PNF）到五细胞期的时间和三细胞期的持续时间。总之，该选择方法被认为是一种可靠的胚胎选择工具[39]。在一项回顾性多中心研究中，分析了 1 664 个 ICSI 周期，其中 799 个周期使用生成算法，865 个周期用于检验其预测值。对受精到二细胞期（t2）、三细胞期（t3）、四细胞期（t4）、五细胞期（t5），以及二细胞维持时长（cc2 = t3 - t2）、三细胞维持时长（s2 = t4 - t3）、种植率、临床妊娠率进行分析，结果显示，t3、cc2、t5 这 3 个参数与种植率相关。根据这些数据，胚胎被分为 4 个亚组。在研究的第二阶段，该算法在 1 620 个移植胚胎中进行了验证，在此阶段，根据该算法对胚胎进行分类，发现不同亚组间的种植率存在显著性差异，认为上述算法是时差成像中胚胎选择的有用工具[40]。

Milevski 等建立了囊胚发育[41]和移植胚胎着床潜能[42]两个预测模型。他们评估了发育到囊胚和未达到囊胚阶段的胚胎之间的胚胎形态动力学参数[41]，以及植入胚胎和非植入胚胎之间的差异[42]。根据研究结果和使用统计分析，生成了 2 个模型，它们将时差成像作为胚胎植入的良好预测工具，但没有囊胚形成模型预测准确性高。

最近，Petersen 等[43]提出了一种适合移植第 3 天胚胎的算法，该算法不依赖于培养条件和受精方法，并回顾性分析了 24 个中心在第 3 天移植的 3 275 个胚胎的记录。新的算法 KIDscore 是基于 6 个时差成像参数开发的，包括 1 个形态学参数和 5 个形态动力学参数，胚胎被分为 5 类，以预测胚胎的着床潜能。该算法通过使用培养至第 5 天的离散胚胎数据集进行验证，以检测其预测囊胚形成的能力。其结论是：KIDscore 可以被认为是一种普遍适用的第三天算法，适用于不同的临床研究[43]。在 884 个 IVF 或 ICSI 周期中观察到 6 种胚胎选择算法（embryo selection algorithms，ESAs）的有效性[15, 40, 44-47]。通过特异性、敏感性、阳性预测值（positive predictive value，PPV）和阴性预测值（negative predictive value，NPV）、受试者工作特征曲线下面积（area under curve，AUC）和每个模型中种植率的概率比（likelihood ratio，LR）来确定每个胚胎选择算法（embryo selection algorithms，ESA）检测胚胎着床潜能的有效性。结果表明，需要根据患者的特点、治疗方案和环境因素来开发预测算法。他们认为，目前的 ESA 在其他诊所应用时可能无法正常工作[48]。Domingez 等[3]结合 TLS 和蛋白质组学，设计了最佳胚胎选择的新模型，他们评估了胚胎培养基中的 7 种蛋白质，并发现了它们与胚胎形态动力学之间的相关性。蛋白质和胚胎时间点之间的最相关参数分别为白细胞介素（IL-6）和 cc2。根据这一关系，他们提出了一种评估胚胎种植率的算法。与其他胚胎参数相比，IL-6 和 cc2（5~12 h）与胚胎种植率具有显著相关性。

目前数据显示，将胚胎形态学变量与关键时间事件相结合，可以生成累积评分模型。这些预测算法整合了不同的变量，但不能较容易地进行调整，难以提供一个全球可接受的模型，因此有必要针对相似患者或条件设计内部模型以实现最优胚胎选择。

1.7 基于时差成像观察的不同研究

时差成像研究的推进为准确研究胚胎发育的过程提供了新方法。时差成像为准确观察早期和晚期胚胎形态动力学，探究胚胎起源、受精方法、遗传异常和观察者差异的相关性提供了可能。下面我们将回顾其中的一些研究。

为了评估治疗相关因素对胚胎形态动力学的影响，我们对243例患者的1 507个胚胎进行了队列研究。结果表明，囊胚期胚胎比卵裂期胚胎更受患者特征影响，患者的年龄和FSH剂量与囊胚发育延迟呈正相关；研究还表明，ICSI受精胚胎第一次卵裂的速度明显快于IVF胚胎[49]。

Minasi等[50]对928个囊胚的形态动力学参数进行了植入前遗传学筛选（PGS）检测，结果显示整倍体和非整倍体胚胎在时差形态动力学方面没有显著差异；同时得出结论，形态动力学参数可以与PGS联合使用，但不能替代PGS用于检测胚胎整倍体状态。但是，另一项回顾性队列研究对时差成像中培养的460个胚胎在第3天进行活检，同时采用比较基因组杂交（comparative genomic hybridization，CGH）芯片检测胚胎非整倍体，结果表明，tPNF、t2、t5、cc2、cc3等动力学参数在正常和非整倍体胚胎中存在显著差异[51]。

关于细胞间通信对胚胎发育的影响，Liu等[52]对765个优质的四细胞期胚胎进行了研究。在受精后第2天，对四细胞期胚胎进行细胞间接触点（intercellular contact point，ICCP）检测，结果显示，与四细胞期结束时达到6个ICCP的胚胎相比，四细胞期结束时少于6个ICCP的胚胎着床潜能降低（5% vs 38.5%）。该研究的结论是：在四细胞期，丢弃形态不良、分裂异常和ICCP少于6个的胚胎，可以显著提高种植率。

为了明确受精方法对胚胎形态动力学的影响，Bodri等[53]回顾性评估了在时差成像中孵育的500个扩张囊胚，结果表明，与ICSI受精的胚胎相比，IVF胚胎在早期胚胎发育阶段（原核消失至t4）明显延迟，而IVF胚胎在囊胚扩张阶段发育更快，常规IVF胚胎和ICSI受精胚胎之间胚胎分裂具有1.5 h的时长差异。然而，明确的结论需要进一步的评估和更多的研究病例支持。

Sundvall等[54]首次评估了观察者间和观察者内部对时间间隔解释的不一致性。3名观察者对158个受精胚胎的时差记录进行了自主解读。结果显示，所有检查参数的相关性都很高，观察者之间的解释非常一致。其中，原核消失的时间、囊胚孵化的完成时间以及第一次分裂后第一个核的出现和消失时间的相关性最高。所有胚胎分裂阶段也近乎一致。二细胞期的多核和均匀性这两个二元参数显示出一致性。观察者内部变异性评估显示大多数参数具有一致性结果。研究指出，胚胎形态动力学因素可准确用于胚胎活力潜能的预测（即使相关情况是由实习员记录的）。

1.8 结论

当前的形态学评估提供的胚胎选择标准不能提高种植率和妊娠率。近年来，基于时差成像的不同研究为胚胎发育提供了新的见解，为胚胎学家提供了改进胚胎评价和选择的方法。对人类胚胎形态动力学的分析可以改善对胚胎分裂早期和晚期胚胎着床潜能及成囊率的预测。时差成像在单胚胎移植（single embryo transfer，SET）政策的进展中发挥了重要作用，可减少多胎妊娠和相关并发症。胚胎时差成像减少了观察者间的差异。远程实现胚胎学判断是时差成像的另一个优点，胚胎学家可以通过互联网在任何地点远程监测胚胎。时差成像也可收集大量数据，包括记录和存储的图像和视频，便于回顾分析。一些研究提出了时差成像的有效结果和临床有效性，但也有其局限性。一方面，对于图像采集过程中胚胎不断暴露于光下（每5～15 min拍摄一张照片），研究人员仍有一些争议。应根据光波长、照明持续时间和成像频率，优先制定胚胎图像捕获指南。同时，胚胎旋转或分裂会影响图像采集，特别是当存在细胞质碎裂或重叠的卵裂球的情况下，视觉观察较困难。另一方面，形态动力学评估对胚胎染色体整倍体状态评估存在限制。众所周知，形态良好的胚胎可能是非整倍体，而次优的胚胎可能是整倍体[21,55]，因此，时差成像应与PGS一起用于检测遗传异常。还有一些混杂因素可能影响时差成像研究中的形态动力学参数，如氧分压、卵巢刺激方案、受精方法、培养基类型、吸烟和高龄等。

最近，一些根据胚胎形态动力学设计的算法提示可预测胚胎着床潜能。这些模型中的时间点是重叠的，当不同实验室应用时，算法可能会失去预测价值。未来需要进行适当设计的研究，以规划具有全球公认的关键时间点和时间间隔的通用算法模型。

总之，种植率应该被视为评估这项新技术成功与否的最终结果。部分研究人员认为，通过时差成像进行胚胎选择仍然是一个实验性的阶段，因为缺乏循证医学来评估这种设备的安全性和有效性。然而，时差成像是一个强大的、无创的用于胚胎发育的研究技术，该技术提供了关于每个胚胎的形态和动态参数信息；同时，应在各个实验室评估该系统的成本效益比，以准确认识该方法的实际有效性。

参考文献

[1] WONG C C, LOEWKE K E, BOSSERT N L, et al. Non-invasive imaging of human embryos before embryonic genome activation predicts development to the blastocyst stage [J]. Nature biotechnology, 2012, 28（10）: 1115-1121.

[2] MESEGUER M, RUBIO I, CRUZ M, et al. Embryo incubation and selection in a time-lapse monitoring system improves pregnancy outcome compared with a standard incubator: a retrospective cohort study [J]. Fertility and sterility, 2012, 98（6）: 1481-1489.

[3] DOMINGUEZ F, MESEGUER M, APARICIO-RUIZ B, et al. New strategy for diagnosing embryo implantation potential by combining proteomics and time-lapse technologies [J]. Fertility and sterility, 2015, 104（4）: 908-914.

[4] ADAMSON G D, ABUSIEF M E, PALAO L, et al. Improved implantation rates of day 3 embryo transfers with the use of an automated time-lapse-enabled test to aid in embryo selection [J]. Fertility and sterility, 2016, 105（2）: 369-375.

[5] KIRKEGAARD K, KESMODEL U S, HINDKJAER J J, et al. Time-lapse parameters as predictors of blastocyst development and pregnancy outcome in embryos from good progno-

sis patients: a prospective cohort study [J]. Human reproduction, 2013, 28 (10): 2643-2651.

[6] MILEWSKI R, CZERNIECKI J, KUCZYNSKA A, et al. Morphokinetic parameters as a source of information concerning embryo developmental and implantation potential [J]. Ginekologia polska, 2016, 87 (10): 677-684.

[7] RUBIO I, GALAN A, LARREATEGUI Z, et al. Clinical validation of embryo culture and selection by morphokinetic analysis: a randomized, controlled trial of the EmbryoScope [J]. Fertility and sterility, 2014, 102 (5): 1287-1294.

[8] DESAI N, PLOSKONKA S, GOODMAN L R, et al. Analysis of embryo morphokinetics, multinucleation and cleavage anomalies using continuous time-lapse monitoring in blastocyst transfer cycles [J]. Reproductive biology and endocrinology: RB&E, 2014, 12: 54.

[9] CONAGHAN J, CHEN A A, WILLMAN S P, et al. Improving embryo selection using a computer-automated time-lapse image analysis test plus day 3 morphology: results from a prospective multicenter trial [J]. Fertility and sterility, 2013, 100 (2): 412-419.

[10] DIAMOND M P, SURAJ V, BEHNKE E J, et al. Using the Eeva Test™ adjunctively to traditional day 3 morphology is informative for consistent embryo assessment within a panel of embryologists with diverse experience [J]. Journal of assisted reproduction and genetics, 2015, 32 (1): 61-68.

[11] HERRERO J, TEJERA A, ALBERT C, et al. A time to look back: analysis of morphokinetic characteristics of human embryo development [J]. Fertility and sterility, 2013, 100 (6): 1602-1609.

[12] MOTATO Y, DE LOS SANTOS M J, ESCRIBA M J, et al. Morphokinetic analysis and embryonic prediction for blastocyst formation through an integrated time-lapse system [J]. Fertility and sterility, 2016, 105 (2): 376-384.

[13] PARK H, BERGH C, SELLESKOG U, et al. No benefit of culturing embryos in a closed system compared with a conventional incubator in terms of number of good quality embryos: results from an RCT [J]. Human reproduction, 2015, 30 (2): 268-275.

[14] NAKAHARA T, IWASE A, GOTO M, et al. Evaluation of the safety of time-lapse observations for human embryos [J]. Journal of assisted reproduction and genetics, 2010, 27 (2-3): 93-96.

[15] CRUZ M, GARRIDO N, HERRERO J, et al. Timing of cell division in human cleavage-stage embryos is linked with blastocyst formation and quality [J]. Reproductive biomedicine online, 2012, 25 (4): 371-381.

[16] KIRKEGAARD K, HINDKJAER J J, GRONDAHL M L, et al. A randomized clinical trial comparing embryo culture in a conventional incubator with a time-lapse incubator [J]. Journal of assisted reproduction and genetics, 2012, 29 (6): 565-572.

[17] WU Y G, LAZZARONI-TEALDI E, WANG Q, et al. Different effectiveness of closed embryo culture system with time-lapse imaging (EmbryoScope™) in comparison to

standard manual embryology in good and poor prognosis patients: A prospectively randomized pilot study [J]. Reproductive biology and endocrinology: RB&E. 2016, 14 (1): 49.

[18] GOODMAN L R, GOLDBERG J, FALCONE T, et al. Does the addition of time-lapse morphokinetics in the selection of embryos for transfer improve pregnancy rates? A randomized controlled trial [J]. Fertility and sterility, 2016, 105 (2): 275 – 285.

[19] ALOMAR M, TASIAUX H, REMACLE S, et al. Kinetics of fertilization and development, and sex ratio of bovine embryos produced using the semen of different bulls [J]. Animal reproduction science, 2008, 107 (1 – 2): 48 – 61.

[20] BERMEJO-ALVAREZ P, ROBERTS R M, ROSENFELD C S. Effect of glucose concentration during in vitro culture of mouse embryos on development to blastocyst, success of embryo transfer, and litter sex ratio [J]. Molecular reproduction and development, 2012, 79 (5): 329 – 336.

[21] ALFARAWATI S, FRAGOULI E, COLLS P, et al. The relationship between blastocyst morphology, chromosomal abnormality, and embryo gender [J]. Fertility and sterility, 2011, 95 (2): 520 – 524.

[22] HENTEMANN M A, BRISKEMYR S, BERTHEUSSEN K. Blastocyst transfer and gender: IVF versus ICSI [J]. Journal of assisted reproduction and genetics, 2009, 26 (8): 433 – 436.

[23] SERDAROGULLARI M, FINDIKLI N, GOKTAS C, et al. Comparison of gender-specific human embryo development characteristics by time-lapse technology [J]. Reproductive biomedicine online, 2014, 29 (2): 193 – 199.

[24] WESTON G, OSIANLIS T, CATT J, et al. Blastocyst transfer does not cause a sex-ratio imbalance [J]. Fertility and sterility, 2009, 92 (4): 1302 – 1305.

[25] BODRI D, KAWACHIYA S, SUGIMOTO T, et al. Time-lapse variables and embryo gender: a retrospective analysis of 81 live births obtained following minimal stimulation and single embryo transfer [J]. Journal of assisted reproduction and genetics, 2016, 33 (5): 589 – 596.

[26] BRONET F, NOGALES M C, MARTÍNEZ E, et al. Is there a relationship between time-lapse parameters and embryo sex? [J]. Fertility and sterility, 2015, 103 (2): 396 – 401.

[27] CHAVEZ S L, LOEWKE K E, HAN J, et al. Dynamic blastomere behaviour reflects human embryo ploidy by the four-cell stage [J]. Nature communications, 2012, 3: 1251.

[28] STENSEN M H, TANBO T G, STORENG R, et al. Fragmentation of human cleavage-stage embryos is related to the progression through meiotic and mitotic cell cycles [J]. Fertility and sterility, 2015, 103 (2): 374 – 381.

[29] REQUENA A, CRUZ M, AGUDO D, et al. Type of gonadotropin during controlled o-

varian stimulation affects the endocrine profile in follicular fluid and apoptosis rate in cumulus cells [J]. European journal of obstetrics, gynecology, and reproductive biology, 2016, 197: 142 - 146.

[30] MUÑOZ M, CRUZ M, HUMAIDAN P, et al. The type of GnRH analogue used during controlled ovarian stimulation influences early embryo developmental kinetics: a time-lapse study [J]. European journal of obstetrics, gynecology, and reproductive biology, 2013, 168 (2): 167 - 172.

[31] GURBUZ A S, GODE F, UZMAN M S, et al. GnRH agonist triggering affects the kinetics of embryo development: a comparative study [J]. Journal of ovarian research, 2016, 9: 22.

[32] MUÑOZ M, CRUZ M, HUMAIDAN P, et al. Dose of recombinant FSH and oestradiol concentration on day of HCG affect embryo development kinetics [J]. Reproductive biomedicine online, 2012, 25 (4): 382 - 389.

[33] MORBECK D E, KRISHER R L, HERRICK J R, et al. Composition of commercial media used for human embryo culture [J]. Fertility and sterility, 2014, 102 (3): 759 - 766.

[34] BASILE N, MORBECK D, GARCÍA-VELASCO J, et al. Type of culture media does not affect embryo kinetics: a time-lapse analysis of sibling oocytes [J]. Human reproduction, 2013, 28 (3): 634 - 641.

[35] HARDARSON T, BUNGUM M, CONAGHAN J, et al. Noninferiority, randomized, controlled trial comparing embryo development using media developed for sequential or undisturbed culture in a time-lapse setup [J]. Fertility and sterility, 2015, 104 (6): 1452 - 1459.

[36] COSTA-BORGÉS N, BELLES M, MESEGUER M, et al. Blastocyst development in single medium with or without renewal on day 3: a prospective cohort study on sibling donor oocytes in a time-lapse incubator [J]. Fertility and sterility, 2016, 105 (3): 707 - 713.

[37] MESEGUER M, HERRERO J, TEJERA A, et al. The use of morphokinetics as a predictor of embryo implantation [J]. Human reproduction, 2011, 26 (10): 2658 - 2671.

[38] FRÉOUR T, LE FLEUTER N, LAMMERS J, et al. External validation of a time-lapse prediction model [J]. Fertility and sterility, 2015, 103 (4): 917 - 922.

[39] LIU Y, CHAPPLE V, FEENAN K, et al. Time-lapse deselection model for human day 3 in vitro fertilization embryos: the combination of qualitative and quantitative measures of embryo growth [J]. Fertility and sterility, 2016, 105 (3): 656 - 662.

[40] BASILE N, VIME P, FLORENSA M, et al. The use of morphokinetics as a predictor of implantation: a multicentric study to define and validate an algorithm for embryo selection [J]. Human reproduction, 2015, 30 (2): 276 - 283.

[41] MILEWSKI R, KUĆ P, KUCZYŃSKA A, et al. A predictive model for blastocyst forma-

tion based on morphokinetic parameters in time-lapse monitoring of embryo development [J]. Journal of assisted reproduction and genetics. 2015, 32 (4): 571-579.

[42] MILEWSKI R, MILEWSKA A J, KUCZYŃSKA A, et al. Do morphokinetic data sets inform pregnancy potential? [J]. Journal of assisted reproduction and genetics. 2016, 33 (3): 357-365.

[43] PETERSEN B M, BOEL M, MONTAG M, et al. Development of a generally applicable morphokinetic algorithm capable of predicting the implantation potential of embryos transferred on day 3 [J]. Human reproduction, 2016, 31 (10): 2231-2244.

[44] AZZARELLO A, HOEST T, MIKKELSEN A L. The impact of pronuclei morphology and dynamicity on live birth outcome after time-lapse culture [J]. Human reproduction, 2012, 27 (9): 2649-2657.

[45] CAMPBELL A, FISHEL S, BOWMAN N, et al. Modelling a risk classification of aneuploidy in human embryos using non-invasive morphokinetics [J]. Reproductive biomedicine online, 2013, 26 (5): 477-485.

[46] CHAMAYOU S, PATRIZIO P, STORACI G, et al. The use of morphokinetic parameters to select all embryos with full capacity to implant [J]. Journal of assisted reproduction and genetics, 2013, 30 (5): 703-710.

[47] DAL CANTO M, COTICCHIO G, MIGNINI RENZINI M, et al. Cleavage kinetics analysis of human embryos predicts development to blastocyst and implantation [J]. Reproductive biomedicine online, 2012, 25 (5): 474-480.

[48] BARRIE A, HOMBURG R, MCDOWELL G, et al. Examining the efficacy of six published time-lapse imaging embryo selection algorithms to predict implantation to demonstrate the need for the development of specific, in-house morphokinetic selection algorithms [J]. Fertility and sterility, 2017, 107 (3): 613-621.

[49] KIRKEGAARD K, SUNDVALL L, ERLANDSEN M, et al. Timing of human preimplantation embryonic development is confounded by embryo origin [J]. Human reproduction, 2016, 31 (2): 324-331.

[50] MINASI M G, COLASANTE A, RICCIO T, et al. Correlation between aneuploidy, standard morphology evaluation and morphokinetic development in 1730 biopsied blastocysts: a consecutive case series study [J]. Human reproduction, 2016, 31 (10): 2245-2254.

[51] CHAWLA M, FAKIH M, SHUNNAR A, et al. Morphokinetic analysis of cleavage stage embryos and its relationship to aneuploidy in a retrospective time-lapse imaging study [J]. Journal of assisted reproduction and genetics, 2015, 32 (1): 69-75.

[52] LIU Y, CHAPPLE V, FEENAN K, et al. Clinical significance of intercellular contact at the four-cell stage of human embryos, and the use of abnormal cleavage patterns to identify embryos with low implantation potential: a time-lapse study [J]. Fertility and sterility, 2015, 103 (6): 1485-1491.

[53] BODRI D, SUGIMOTO T, SERNA J Y, et al. Influence of different oocyte insemination

techniques on early and late morphokinetic parameters: retrospective analysis of 500 time-lapse monitored blastocysts [J]. Fertility and sterility, 2015, 104 (5): 1175 – 1181.

[54] SUNDVALL L, INGERSLEV H J, BRETH KNUDSEN U, et al. Inter-and intra-observer variability of time-lapse annotations [J]. Human reproduction, 2013, 28 (12): 3215 – 3221.

[55] ZIEBE S, LUNDIN K, LOFT A, et al. FISH analysis for chromosomes 13, 16, 18, 21, 22, X and Y in all blastomeres of IVF pre-embryos from 144 randomly selected donated human oocytes and impact on pre-embryo morphology [J]. Human reproduction, 2003, 18 (12): 2575 – 2581.

(Nasim Tabibnejad)

第 4 章 体外胚胎分裂的时空分析方法

在胚胎分裂阶段,对早期胚胎进行图像自动或半自动时差分析,可以深入了解有丝分裂的时间变化,胚胎和细胞谱系的分裂时间和分裂模式的规律。同时,监测胚胎发育的分子变迁过程可以研究基因表达与细胞生理和发育之间的联系。胚胎的四维视频分析会产生大量数据,这不仅对具有生理活性的胚胎研究的硬件和胚胎保存的设备提出了新的要求,同时还间接地对分析软件和数据分析处理提出了新的要求。通过研究形态动力学和形态学,连续拍摄和自动分析生长中胚胎,可以为预测胚胎发育潜能提供新见解。这些技术直到最近几年才得以高效实现,在此之前都是通过烦琐的手动过程得以实现。近年来,已经开发了几种方法来实现对活胚胎的动态监测。本章描述了三种不同的硬件和软件分析方法,并给出了结果示例。胚胎及其谱系分裂模式是在体内研究实现的,这些方法可为发育胚胎学的探索打开一扇新窗户。

尽管经过 30 多年(截至目前已有 40 多年——编者注)的实践,体外受精(IVF)中胚胎植入子宫的成功率仍然只有 30% 左右(不同年龄段和不同地区的患者的成功率有差异)[1-2]。因此,当选择体外培养的胚胎并将其植入子宫时,选择质量最好的胚胎是至关重要的。这不仅将提高活产率,而且还将减少多胚胎移植,从而降低双胎妊娠和新生儿并发症的风险,也能减少母亲妊娠相关的健康问题。尽管培养方法有所改进,但目前胚胎选择仍然主要基于形态学标准的人工评估,其中在识别与胚胎发育相关的形态学特征方面已进行了大量研究。基因筛查和培养基代谢谱等其他方法是否能提高妊娠率,目前存在争议[3-9]。对于形态学在胚胎质量评估中的相关性,目前还在讨论中[10],它很可能在未来的 IVF 胚胎评估中继续发挥重要作用。以往,胚胎质量评估是通过在胚胎发育的间歇时间点使用光学显微镜进行手动检查;最近,新的技术解决方案使得利用时差成像连续监测胚胎成为可能,为基于动态特性的胚胎评估开辟了新的可能性。

在记录期结束时具有相似形态外观的胚胎之间,胚胎内关键事件发生的时间可能会有很大差异,并且胚胎形态可能在数小时内发生变化[11-14],说明动态监测胚胎优于间歇监测。胚胎研究的一个重要终点是胚胎分裂的时间,这已被证实与胚胎活力和着床潜能相关[15-18]。出于研究目的,追踪早期胚胎中的细胞谱系和细胞定位为理解胚胎多能性提供了重要信息。胚胎也是研究发育生物学和三维细胞相互作用的良好模型。连续拍摄和分析生长中的胚胎的发育潜能,研究形态动力学和形态学,为胚胎发育提供了新的

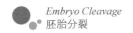

见解。过去胚胎发育潜能的预测只能通过烦琐的手动过程才能实现。尽管目前一些人类 IVF 实验室已经开始使用时差成像技术来监测胚胎的分裂和生长,但还需要对该技术及其潜能进行进一步的描述或分析。本章的重点是研究随时间变化的具有活性的早期胚胎的方法,以及它们作为胚胎学研究和临床应用的新工具的可能性。

1 活体成像在胚胎学中的作用

传统的显微镜有诸多缺点,如需要固定样品、只能间歇地提供静态信息。由于在静态分析中,大多数关于细胞对环境的反应、动态基因表达和时间的信息都会丢失,因此,对细胞分裂和发育的全面理解需要从单个细胞水平上的动态视角去观察。近年来,活体成像技术为显微镜、样品处理以及单个细胞活体成像的硬件和软件提供了新的工具。在活细胞中有几个单细胞和单分子监测的例子,可使用基于分子标记或无标记的方法研究早期胚胎的发育[19-22]。

荧光标记能够追踪特定蛋白质并测量其特性,以研究基因表达、蛋白质定位与功能以及蛋白质间的相互作用。通过同时使用多个标记,可以同时跟踪多个蛋白质或基因的表达。借助时差显微镜,细胞内事件可以与细胞间相互作用和最终细胞命运等外部因素联系起来。这些方法使我们对基因表达、细胞相互作用和异质过程的动力学有了全新的认识。在荧光成像中,激光用于激发特定波长的荧光团。当荧光标记在返回其未激发的分子状态时发光时,可以使用全场外延荧光来测量光[23]。在共焦成像中,引入针孔与聚焦激光相结合,可有效降低背景荧光,并允许通过机械扫描对样品进行光学切片。改变针孔大小将有效地改变被成像样品的厚度、图像分辨率和采集时间。

对于某些应用,使用荧光标记是不可行的。通过连续拍摄胚胎材料,可以从时差序列中提取细胞轮廓、位置、形状和纹理等重要信息,而无须使用荧光标记。通过匹配和跟踪,这些信息可以结合到分裂胚胎的时间分布图中,检测分裂的时间并跟踪细胞谱系。将计算机视觉与无创成像方法相结合,可以在样本干扰最小的情况下连续研究胚胎生长。荧光成像允许对基因表达和细胞内特征进行无创性测量,而无标记光学显微镜允许跟踪随时间变化的细胞大小、形状和行为,以响应分子变化。这种结合使我们有可能直接监测细胞反应和基因表达变化对环境的反应。建立一个细胞模型,可以将分子尺度连接到细胞尺度,映射出化学世界和生物世界之间的实际联系。

2 胚胎成像的无创技术

目前已有一种生物技术成功应用于小鼠和人类的胚胎成像,该技术包括添加荧光标记和无标记两种方法。出于研究目的,如果使用的方案不会显著干扰胚胎生长,则添加荧光蛋白(fluorescent proteins,FP),这是一种无创方法。在人类胚胎学的临床应用中,不能使用任何类型的标记物。这里我们将荧光标记方法称为无创方法,并将"真正"的无创方法指定为"无标记"。

2.1 荧光成像

添加荧光蛋白是选择性研究特定细胞内靶点的标准方法[24]。最常见的荧光标签是源自水母 *Aeqourea victoria* 的绿色荧光蛋白[25-26]。FP 是通过质粒 DNA 表达载体的转染或微量注射引入的,该载体携带蛋白质的遗传密码。通过用 FP 标记感兴趣的生物功能蛋白,可以跟踪特定的途径。FPs 的使用提供了一种在细胞内定位蛋白质的简单方法,但该方法也有缺点,在足够短的波长和较高的激光激发强度下可能产生光毒性[27]。此外,FP 的瞬时表达可能导致伴随它的功能蛋白水平高于正常水平,这可能对整个系统的动态行为产生不可预见的影响;或可使用靶向基因组编辑技术(如 CRISPR-Cas9)将 FP 整合到基因组中,在这种情况下,每个细胞的质粒拷贝数将不再影响蛋白质浓度。对照实验对于确定 FP 研究方法的效果是必要的,但对于每个研究系统或实验环境需要区别对待。

测定还可以通过荧光漂白恢复(fluorescence recovery after photobleaching,FRAP)来研究 FP 结合位点周围的动力学[28]。在 FRAP 中,荧光团共价连接到感兴趣的分子,随后使用特定波长的入射激光辐照漂白荧光团。随着新的荧光团迁移到该区域,可以通过研究光漂白斑点的逐渐变亮来量化分子的扩散。三种密切相关的技术是光漂白中的荧光损失(the fluorescence loss in photobleaching,FLIP)、光活化后的荧光衰减(fluorescence decay after photoactivation,FDAP)和荧光相关光谱(fluorescence correlation spectroscopy,FCS)[29]。荧光共振能量转移(fluorescence resonance energy transfer,FRET)[有时也称为弗尔斯特(Förster)共振能量转移]可用于研究蛋白质-蛋白质相互作用[30]。入射激光将供体荧光团置于激发状态,并且将激发分子状态下保持的能量转移到非常接近(通常小于 10 nm)的受体荧光团。当研究中的 2 个分子分别用供体和受体荧光团标记时,从受体荧光团检测到的光表明这 2 个分子非常接近。

目前已有许多研究使用荧光标记的各种成像方式研究胚胎内或胚胎干细胞的蛋白质运动[31-36]。

2.2 无标记显微镜

目前,IVF 中心或诊所正在使用的两种主要的胚胎成像技术是霍夫曼调制对比成像(Hoffman modulation contrast imaging,HMC)(有时称为白光)[37-38]和暗场成像(darkfield imaging,DF)[39]。出于研究目的,相干反斯托克斯拉曼散射(coherent anti-Stokes Raman scattering,CARS)[40]和光学显微镜[41]的使用也变得越来越普遍。在 IVF 胚胎的时差成像开始使用之前,HMC 是标准的且仍用于手动显微镜的成像技术。时差成像得到的图像与胚胎学家惯用的显微镜图像相似,因此,对于比较手动和计算机自动注释图像来说,后者是一个优势。HMC 最适合用于细胞内部细节的成像。另外,暗场为细膜等边缘结构提供了更好的细节，并能更准确地检测和跟踪细胞轮廓。

暗场成像是一种排除任何未散射光的成像方法，使样品在较暗的背景上显得更亮，并增强成像和未染色样品的对比度[42]。这是一种简单而有效的无创增强样品对比度的方法，但其缺点是可供采集的光线较弱。为了进行补偿，必须对样品进行强光照射，但强光照射可能导致样品损坏。然而，低亮度也意味着图像几乎完全没有光学伪影。暗场显微镜在研究折射率差异较大的边界结构时最为有用，例如，用于细胞膜的成像比内部细胞结构更为有效。它最适合折射率差异较大的薄样品（如有锐利边缘的样品），而对于厚样品可能会出现伪影。

HMC 成像是霍夫曼在 1975 年发明的[43]。如今，它是一种常用的生物样品无创对比增强技术。它的优点是对比度好、曝光量低、分辨率高、景深短，可在物镜数值孔径控制的分辨率下进行聚焦剖切。样品均匀性会影响切片效果。其缺点为强烈的光学伪影和不适合计算机图像处理的图像外观。HMC 通常用于胚胎学研究，目前在许多商业产品中已经使用。

3　活胚胎成像的挑战

尽管近年来活体单细胞成像技术取得了进展，但其在更广泛的应用方面仍存在一些挑战。长期成像和分析的实验不仅须确保高质量成像，还须确保长期支持样本活力和适当的分析计算方法。体外观察胚胎需要一个培养箱环境，以便在成像期间提供最佳的生存条件或样本条件。温度变化会影响生理过程的功能以及反应动力学，并且随着研究时长增加，挑战会增大。一种解决方案是在显微镜上安装培养流动室，减少气体和培养液的量，以将样品维持在小体积；但这种方案存在缺点，即培养室表面有出现冷凝的风险。另一种方法是将显微镜光学系统集成到培养箱中，这要求显微镜光学系统和电子系统在潮湿、温和的环境中工作。还有少量的商业解决方案，这些解决方案将胚胎孵化与成像硬件相结合。使用这些解决方案时，胚胎培养基和容器不得在光路中引入成像伪影，如光反射表面、自动荧光或过大的培养基体积。另一个挑战是从孵育处装载和回收细胞的过程可能导致细胞识别丢失。对于 IVF，培养箱和显微镜存在多种组合[44]，可以是集成解决方案，也可以是设计用于培养箱内的新显微镜。到目前为止，在标准间歇式培养箱系统和时差培养箱系统中培养的胚胎的生长和种植率没有差异[45-47]。一项研究发现，时差组的流产率较高，应谨慎使用；但该方式对植入胚胎的妊娠率或胚胎健康没有影响[48]。

在非人类 IVF 中，通常使用相差显微镜代替 HMC。相差显微镜与 HMC 相似，因为它提供了高水平的图像细节，但样品物体周围有以光晕形式出现的图像伪影。不同物种胚胎的不同外观将影响使用哪种光学系统。一些物种的胚胎颜色较深、致密（如猪），而另一些物种的胚胎则较半透明（如小鼠）。因此，不同物种胚胎的最佳光学系统各不相同，必须相应地选择合适的分析软件。使用暗场成像的单细胞研究受硬件限制，仅限于四细胞期至六细胞期。在 HMC 中使用局部剖片，可以对从合子到囊胚期的整个胚胎进行成像，但随着细胞数量的增加，自动分析变得越来越困难。因为尽管进行了切片，但无法去除失焦图像的细节。在人类 IVF 中，八细胞期之前是自动检测的一个可行阶段，九细胞期至十六细胞期的致密化会降低细胞边界的可视性。空泡化和囊胚形成阶段也为图像的自动分析提供了机会，包括囊胚的扩张和塌陷事件。

在非人类哺乳动物胚胎的荧光时差成像中，荧光团的寿命是有限的，这种效应称为光漂白[27]。光漂白可以通过减少曝光来限制，但最终会限制胚胎成像的持续时间。其中最严重的问题是胚胎长时间暴露在强激光下引起的毒性效应。这种光毒性可以通过使用机械快速快门或开关 LED 最小化激光照射改善，但任何快门都会在连续时差成像装置中快速达到其寿命的终点。以 1 Hz 的频率切换为例，快门将在大约 12 天内打开和关闭 100 万次，因此需要一个高效的显微镜控制软件。

在收集的信息和潜在样本有害暴露之间需要做出取舍，必须根据研究终点和所研究动态的预期频率仔细选择图像捕获频率。在同时监测多个样本的情况下，存在两种解决方案：其一，在每次扫描图像捕获时，移动并重新定位成像硬件或样本。在这种情况下，在成像的样本和每个样本捕获的图像之间存在权衡（受移动力学的限制）。其二，在全场扫描时，捕获的图像同时包含所有样本。在这种情况下，取而代之的是在成像的样本数量和每个样本可用的图像分辨率之间进行权衡。

对于二维成像，全场技术是最有效的，因为它们在一次曝光中捕获了整个视野。然而，随着时间推移、序列长度的增加，系统的稳定性变得至关重要。焦点漂移是一个主要问题，需要一种自动对焦机制或一种用户输入校正方法。

即使捕获频率适中，特别是数据如果以多维度和成像方式同时记录的话，时差研究的数据量也可能迅速增加到 TB 甚至更多。因此，必须考虑数据存储、分析数据的有效访问以及采集后分析需求。少量的视频数据可以手动分析，但这种方法很快变得烦琐和耗时，因此需要使用自动或半自动方法进行分析。手动评估图像容易出现不同观察者之间可变性的错误[49-50]。在图像捕获阶段考虑预期的分析，可以提前优化采集图像质量和硬件设置。目前有多种用于视频序列分析的开源软件应用程序，然而它们通常不适合对多维数据进行更高级的分析，而这在胚胎研究中都是经常需要的。在胚胎研究中，三维扫描或焦点切片可用于捕获多维数据。与通用应用程序相比，为数据量身定制的专用解决方案通常速度更快、精度更高。底层真实情况的注释图像数据的获取决定了分析工具的开发。随着生成的图像数据量的增加，此类训练数据的可用性已成为一个显著的瓶颈。现有的解决方案增加了数据和注释的共享和开放访问，这需要数据管理、格式和元数据存储的标准化方法。为此，开放源代码的生物图像数据库系统（如 Offline Message Editor Remote Objects，OMERO[51]）是一个重要的途径。

分析的最佳选择因实验设置和研究目的不同而大不相同。通常，最初的分析步骤是识别图像中的细胞轮廓。在胚胎成像中，有多种检测和跟踪细胞轮廓的方法，既有基于分割的方法（需要识别胚胎细胞轮廓），也有无分割的方法[52-55]，或这些方法的组合[56]。通常，正确执行的分割[54,57-59]提供了有关细胞位置、形状和轮廓的最详细信息，但在计算上也更具挑战性。

目前尚无一套长期成像的实验条件可以普遍应用于各类场景。每个生物学问题和模型都需要其特定的硬件和软件工具组合，且需要定制。这些挑战的解决方案将使未来胚胎学的重大发现成为可能。Kang 等[60]和 Turksen 等[61]分别提供了荧光标记与干细胞成像及追踪的有用总结。以下举例说明人类和非人类胚胎的成功的时差成像方法，以及使用三种不同的方法解决实验挑战的途径。

4 方法1：使用荧光标记的三维小鼠胚胎形态

为了解分裂期胚胎细胞的致密化、细胞谱系、细胞重排和动态行为，动态成像是必要的。本方法研究了丝状体形成在胚胎致密化、顶端收缩、多能干细胞内化和胚胎致密化前细胞定位中的作用，这些被认为是胚胎细胞多能发育的重要因素。此外，可使用多种靶向荧光标记的蛋白质和转录因子监测细胞内的过程。

可以利用荧光显微镜选择性地激发和显示 FP 作为活组织中的标记。基因编码 FP 的发现允许对大多数细胞蛋白质进行包括监测其分布和动态在内的定量分析[62]。由于需要在体内研究胚胎发育，因此荧光成像成为一种完美解决观察胚胎发育问题的技术。与宽场荧光成像相反，使用共聚焦显微镜时，探测器针孔阻挡了聚焦区域外的荧光[63]，这使得共聚焦成像能够减少宽场荧光显微镜引起的一些散射效应。然而，扫描单个截面意味着激发，因此会破坏焦平面上方和下方的离焦区域。此外，针孔还将排除从焦平面发射的散射信号光子，因为它们会远离检测样本。因此，宽场和共聚焦成像是最适合于厚度小于 40 μm 的薄样品的方法。为了研究在直径约 100 μm（70% 细胞部分加透明带）的小鼠胚胎中发生的相关事件，需要使用双光子激发（two-photon excitation，2PE）荧光显微镜。

双光子激发荧光显微镜是一种在高分辨率和对比度下限制样品光毒性并延长成像时间和深度的方法[64]。在 2PE 中，需要 2 个一半激发能量的光子才能将 FP 置于激发态。在 2PE 中使用激光产生聚焦在焦平面区域的更高强度，这可使激发能量限制在非常小的体积内（通常约为 0.1 μm³）。共聚焦显微镜和 2PE 荧光显微镜的组合可用于跟踪和表征发育中胚胎的不同形态变化，如细胞分裂、极性、丝状体形成和动力学、致密化和囊胚空化（图 4-1）。因此，使用特定的荧光标记蛋白质或肽标记细胞核、细胞质或细胞膜成分，可优化共聚焦和 2PE 荧光成像方法[29, 31, 65]。允许以小于 60 s 的间隔扫描单个胚胎，并使用 Imaris（Bitplane AG）或 ZEN（蔡司）软件重建三维胚胎形态。长期拍照定位软件（蔡司 ZEN）可用于成像 20～30 个相邻培养的胚胎（图 4-1）。得益于共聚焦显微镜和 2PE 荧光显微镜的高灵敏度探测器，长期成像可以持续 24 h 以上而不会影响小鼠胚胎的健康和完整性。因此，可以对 20～30 个胚胎中进行过夜的细胞动力学成像拍摄。从八细胞期到囊胚期（间隔约 36 h），每隔 40 min 拍摄一次图像。利用明场光学系统捕获荧光成像，可以同时监测细胞和分子动力学变化（图 4-1D）。

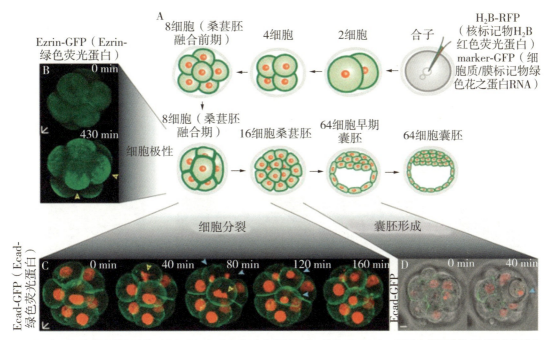

A. 在一细胞期注射细胞核（H_2B-RFP）和细胞质或膜标记物（标记物 GFP），显示小鼠胚胎发育过程中的形态发生变化；B. 细胞极性事件（箭头）在 Ezrin-GFP 蛋白显示的八细胞期观察到；C. 使用膜标记物 Ecad GFP 和核标记物 H_2B-RFP 监测胞质分裂和细胞分裂时间，染色质凝聚用虚线箭头突出显示，细胞分裂用普通箭头突出显示；D. 用明场光学结合膜和核标记物的荧光成像（Ecad GFP 和 H_2B-RFP）观察胚泡形成过程中的空泡化（箭头）。比例尺 = 10 μm。

图 4-1　小鼠胚胎发育

研究从合子到囊胚期亚细胞标记物的动态，可以开展不同发育阶段蛋白质的亚细胞定位研究。为实现该实验目的，使用 pCS2+表达载体[66]和合成加帽修饰的 RNA（使用 Ambion mMessage mMachine SP6 转录试剂盒），将加帽标记 GFP RNA 注射到单细胞期胚胎中。对于细胞核，H_2B-RFP 通常用作标记物，而 memb-mCherry、Ecad-RFP、Ecad-GFP 或 Ezrin-RFP 可用于细胞膜的监测（图 4-1）[32, 34, 65]。图 4-1C 为使用核标记物 H_2B-GFP 和膜标记物 Ecad-GFP 的示例。细胞极性事件可用 Ezrin-GFP 进行研究。Ezrin 在胚胎致密化过程中极化之前在所有细胞中均表达[67]（图 4-1B）。因此，与 Ezrin-GFP 共定位是研究任何感兴趣的蛋白质在致密化和细胞极性过程中的动力学和分布的极好方法。

5　方法2：使用机器学习对人类胚胎进行细胞谱系研究

本方法侧重于在胚胎的暗场时差显微镜图像中自动监测人类胚胎细胞，目的是开发在每个时间节点上用于区分、检测、定位胚胎细胞的方法，并对完整过程进行细胞谱系分析。这一方法为胚胎学家和体外受精临床医生了解人类胚胎的发育和更准确地选择发育潜能胚胎提供了一个有用的工具。

与其他细胞（如干细胞和其他物种的胚胎细胞）不同，非染色人类胚胎细胞的自动分析面临复杂的发育模式的挑战，如胚胎紧凑生长和细胞重叠。由于暗场成像模式单平面成像的限制，非染色人类胚胎细胞的致密度变化和深度信息发生丢失。

自动化分析重要的第一步是能够从背景噪声中高效、可靠地分割胚胎。为此，通过分割定义一个能量最小化问题并通过图形切割解决，开发一个通过估计胚胎周围轮廓来分割发育中胚胎的框架[68]。其次，细胞在空间上被定位并随后被检测到分裂。为便于定位，将建模单元定义为适合每个时间段椭圆的轮廓（图4-2）。

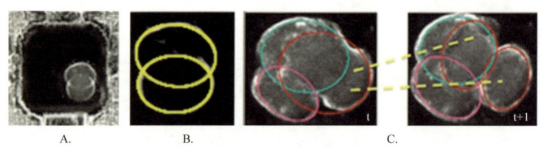

A. 双细胞期人类胚胎的暗场显微镜图像示例；B. 拟合椭圆的细胞定位；C. 用于谱系树构建的3～4个细胞分裂关联图。

图4-2 非染色人类胚胎细胞在暗场中的成像模式

预测细胞数量是细胞生物学分析中的一项基本任务，也是定位胚胎卵裂事件的一种间接方法。细胞数量在人类胚胎发育中是最重要的，因为目前的胚胎活力生物标志物需要精确的细胞计数。可以直接从显微镜图像[69]或通过检测（定位）细胞[70-71]来预测细胞数量，两者也可以结合使用。本方法即是在条件随机场（conditional random field，CRF）[72]中结合使用了上述两者来预测细胞数量。其结果是通过记录相邻帧之间的细胞关联来建立细胞分裂早期模型，从而形成时差序列的完整谱系树。细胞谱系分析在了解胚胎发育动力学方面至关重要，是细胞生物学分析的基本步骤。细胞谱系树和分段形状现在可以用于研究生长胚胎的各种属性，如细胞分裂的时间、异常分裂模式和细胞对称性（图4-3）。

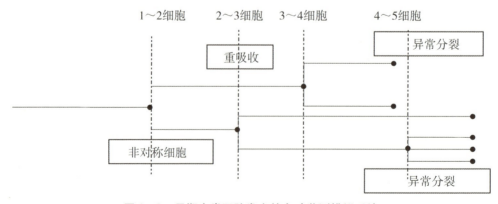

图4-3 早期人类胚胎发育的自动监测模拟系统

6 方法3：使用视频图像处理的人类胚胎分析

当涉及人类胚胎的图像细节时，HMC 成像具有优越性，然而，由光学调制引入的光学伪影会导致边缘结构多个梯度出现。对焦对象通常清晰可见，但来自对焦对象的叠加光通常会在图像中引入"阴影"。该方法没有荧光标记细胞，其结果是细胞轮廓分割困难，但细胞内部结构的细节展示程度很高。可以尝试分割该图像，但后续分析通常取决于分割后轮廓的清晰程度，因此该方法易引入累积误差。该方法的重点是检测胚胎中与发育相关的事件，如致密化、囊胚腔形成、细胞核定位、细胞分裂和胚胎碎片，因此对于胚胎图片无须完全分割。

原始图像在空间上叠加得到胚胎对应位置，并从胚胎内部提取一组图像特征[73-74]。随着胚胎的生长，图像的特征也会发生改变，从而可以在没有完整图像数据的情况下描绘胚胎发育的轮廓[75]。图4-4 显示胚胎内部图像的灰度变化用于绘制二维胚胎发育状态。灰度变化是图像对比度的一种度量，每个细胞分裂会引入一个新的细胞，从而在图像中引入一组新的较暗的细胞膜，每个细胞分裂都会增加灰度变化，从而导致图像灰度变化的增加。因此，每个细胞分裂事件都可以被检测为方差分布中的两侧突然变陡坡时刻。当细胞膜变得不那么明显时，胚胎致密化被检测为大量的变异损失，随后随着胚胎形成囊胚腔，变异又增加。随着时间的推移，胚胎的理想发育遵循一种可预测的模式，与直接使用图像相比，卵裂等事件更容易被自动检测到（图4-4），而异常发育事件将明显不同于正常发育事件（图4-5）。

当图像的高度细节可以展示时，为了进行特征检测，细胞核和原核等细胞内结构也可以进行分割（图4-6）。分割区域在形状和大小上受到限制，我们需要确保定位的结构具有预定义的生物学形状。以旋转的形式引入轻微干扰，可有效地平均定位结构并防止检测误报[74]。使用一个框架，从合子到囊胚的整个发育过程都可以被描绘出来，并与相关的细胞内隔室（如细胞核）的可见性相结合，而该过程不需要任何荧光标记。

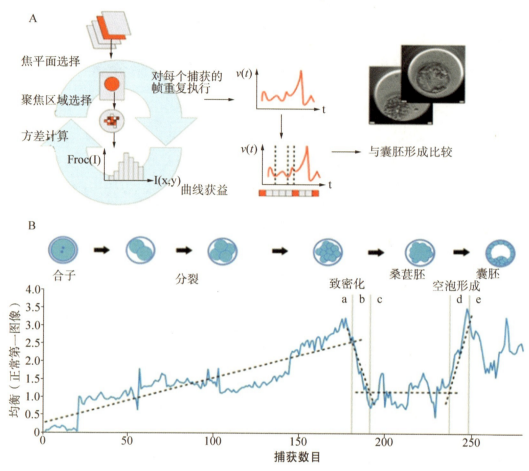

A. 胚胎捕获图像的计算管线示意。从图像堆栈中选择最佳焦平面。在每个单独的图像中选择一个感兴趣区域，并为每个区域计算一个图像强度方差值。对图像序列中的每次捕获图片重复此过程，得到一个函数$v(t)$，将方差描述为时间的函数。然后进一步分析$v(t)$是否出现可检测的关键事件，并对胚胎发育进行分析。最后，对形成囊胚的胚胎和未形成囊胚的胚胎进行比较。B. 胚胎在280帧捕获过程中的图像强度变化，标准化为序列中的第一幅图像。胚胎分裂阶段的分裂可检测为图像方差的突然增加，由卵裂球经历有丝分裂，图像中的边缘数量增加所致。在致密化开始时，单个卵裂球膜不再可区分，变异性下降，在桑葚胚期保持在较低水平。如果在囊胚阶段，胚胎表现出几次塌陷和再膨胀周期，随着囊胚腔扩张组可能发生剧烈波动，差异再次增加。胚胎的生长分为5个阶段：a. 最初的分裂从受精到开始致密化；b. 开始致密化到完成致密化；c. 桑葚胚；d. 空泡化；e. 囊胚。计算了每个截面的平均值和方差变化。虚线趋势线说明变化过程[75]。

图4-4 胚胎成像示意

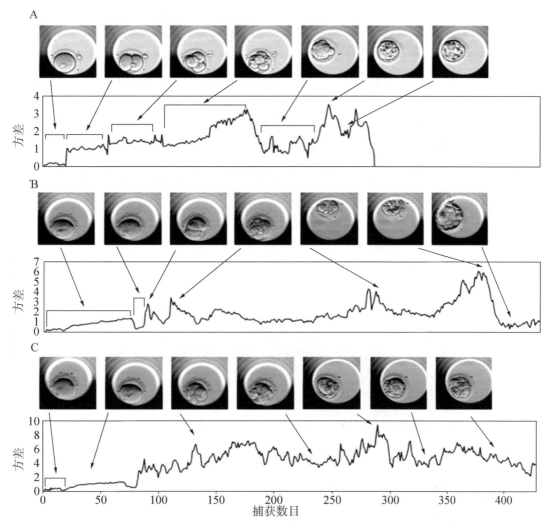

方差是根据围绕胚胎中心的圆形区域的图像强度计算得到的。在方差剖面中可以看到特征变化的点上显示了一些示例图像。A. 质量好的胚胎，有丝分裂是图像方差连续增加，桑葚胚期是方差降低的时期；B. 清晰看到原核破裂，即使最终形成囊胚，但在胚胎分裂阶段形成较多的细胞碎片；C. 原核破裂明显，胚胎发育早期出现细胞碎片，未形成囊胚[75]。

图4-5　胚胎质量依次下降的3个代表性胚胎的轮廓

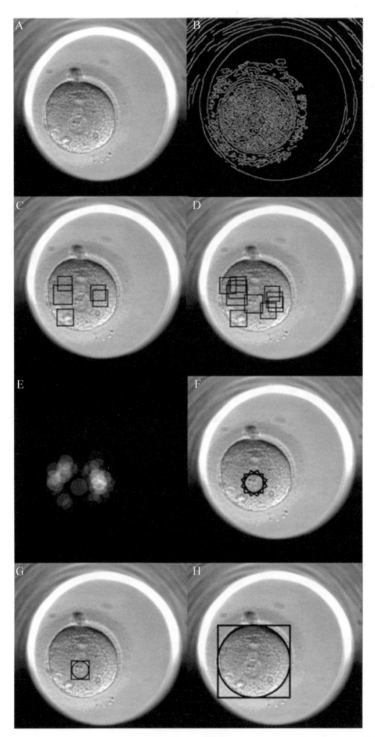

A. 原始图像;B. 边缘检测;C. 选择 5 个最重要的圆形结构;D. 选择 10 个最重要的圆形结构;E. 从同一图像中选择的圆形结构重叠旋转 60°;F. 原核轮廓显示,以不同角度进行 3 次计算的重叠;G. 选择原核的轮廓;H. 所选合子的轮廓[74]。

图 4-6　人类胚胎中合子和原核的检测

7 结论

研究证明,胚胎可以在子宫外生长14天以上,14天也是法律规定的体外培养的限制时限[76]。由于体外培养技术的限制,有关早期胚胎发育时期的研究还很少。通过软件分析、成像和孵化器技术的新组合等从全新角度研究胚胎发育将会成为可能。

通过对细胞核和质膜使用特定的FP标记蛋白标记,可以跟踪哺乳动物胚胎发育过程中重要形态发生变化的动力学特征,包括囊胚形成过程中的细胞分裂、细胞极性和空泡化。使用诸如基因沉默(敲除)、过表达或使用所选基因抑制剂阻断等技术,这些发育特征的定量分析为功能和表型研究的设计铺平了道路。这些方法的组合可为发育功能和疾病提供重要见解。

体内胚胎的自动或半自动无标记分析方法使研究胚胎发育的时间比以前更长成为现实,从而为人类胚胎早期发育开辟了一套新的方法(其中伦理因素对研究方法的选择非常重要)。通过对IVF中常规生长的胚胎进行时差摄像研究,可以在临床环境中收集研究数据,同时这些方法也有助于更好地监测IVF胚胎。

总之,这些无创方法为增加对一般发育胚胎学以及特定医学问题(如胚胎分裂模式、谱系和人类低生育率背后的原因)的理解打开了一扇窗口。

致谢

Anna Leida Mölder 感谢曼彻斯特大都会大学的帮助和支持。Juan Carlos Fierro-González 感谢瑞典医学研究学会提供的支持。

参考文献

[1] DIAMOND M P, WILLMAN S, CHENETTE P, et al. The clinical need for a method of identification of embryos destined to become a blastocyst in assisted reproductive technology cycles [J]. Journal of assisted reproduction and genetics, 2012, 29 (5): 391-396.

[2] European IVF-Monitoring Consortium (EIM), European Society of Human Reproduction and Embryology (ESHRE), KUPKA M S, et al. Assisted reproductive technology in Europe, 2011: results generated from European registers by ESHRE [J]. Human reproduction, 2016, 31 (2): 233-248.

[3] HARDARSON T, AHLSTRÖM A, ROGBERG L, et al. Non-invasive metabolomic profiling of Day 2 and 5 embryo culture medium: a prospective randomized trial [J]. Human reproduction, 2012, 27 (1): 89-96.

[4] MASTENBROEK S, TWISK M, VAN ECHTEN-ARENDS J, et al. In vitro fertilization with preimplantation genetic screening [J]. The New England journal of medicine, 2007,

357（1）：9-17.
[5] VERGOUW C G, KIESLINGER D C, KOSTELIJK E H, et al. Metabolomic profiling of culture media by near infrared spectroscopy as an adjunct to morphology for selection of a single day 3 embryo to transfer in IVF：a double-blind randomised trial［J］. Fertility and sterility, 2011, 96（3）：S3.
[6] OTTOSEN L D M, HINDKJAER J, INGERSLEV J. Light exposure of the ovum and pre-implantation embryo during ART procedures［J］. Journal of assisted reproduction and genetics, 2007, 24（2-3）：99-103.
[7] JONES G M, CRAM D S, SONG B, et al. Novel strategy with potential to identify developmentally competent IVF blastocysts［J］. Human reproduction, 2008, 23（8）：1748-1759.
[8] SCOTT L, BERNTSEN J, DAVIES D, et al. Symposium：innovative techniques in human embryo viability assessment. Human oocyte respiration-rate measurement：potential to improve oocyte and embryo selection?［J］. Reproductive biomedicine online, 2008, 17（4）：461-469.
[9] SELI E, ROBERT C, SIRARD M A. OMICS in assisted reproduction：possibilities and pitfalls［J］. Molecular human reproduction, 2010, 16（8）：513-530.
[10] HARDARSON T, CAISANDER G, SJÖGREN A, et al. A morphological and chromosomal study of blastocysts developing from morphologically suboptimal human pre-embryos compared with control blastocysts［J］. Human reproduction, 2003, 18（2）：399-407.
[11] MONTAG M, LIEBENTHRON J, KÖSTER M. Which morphological scoring system is relevant in human embryo development?［J］. Placenta, 2011, 32（Suppl 3）：S252-S256.
[12] VAN BLERKOM J, DAVIS P, ALEXANDER S. A microscopic and biochemical study of fragmentation phenotypes in stage-appropriate human embryos［J］. Human reproduction, 2001, 16（4）：719-729.
[13] LEMMEN J G, AGERHOLM I, ZIEBE S. Kinetic markers of human embryo quality using time-lapse recordings of IVF/ICSI-fertilized oocytes［J］. Reproductive biomedicine online, 2008, 17（3）：385-391.
[14] ALIKANI M, COHEN J, TOMKIN G, et al. Human embryo fragmentation in vitro and its implications for pregnancy and implantation［J］. Fertility and sterility, 1999, 71（5）：836-842.
[15] CRUZ M, GARRIDO N, HERRERO J, et al. Timing of cell division in human cleavage-stage embryos is linked with blastocyst formation and quality［J］. Reproductive biomedicine online, 2012, 25（4）：371-381.
[16] CHEN A A, TAN L, SURAJ V, et al. Biomarkers identified with time-lapse imaging：discovery, validation, and practical application［J］. Fertility and sterility, 2013, 99

(4): 1035 – 1043.

[17] HLINKA D, KAL'ATOVÁ B, UHRINOVÁ I, et al. Time-lapse cleavage rating predicts human embryo viability [J]. Physiological research, 2012, 61 (5): 513 – 525.

[18] MESEGUER M, HERRERO J, TEJERA A, et al. The use of morphokinetics as a predictor of embryo implantation [J]. Human reproduction, 2011, 26 (10): 2658 – 2671.

[19] SATO S, RANCOURT A, SATO Y, et al. Single-cell lineage tracking analysis reveals that an established cell line comprises putative cancer stem cells and their heterogeneous progeny [J]. Scientific reports, 2016, 6: 23328.

[20] VAN VALEN D A, KUDO T, LANE K M, et al. Deep learning automates the quantitative analysis of individual cells in live-cell imaging experiments [J]. PLoS computational biology, 2016, 12 (11): e1005177.

[21] LLAMOSI A, GONZALEZ-VARGAS A M, VERSARI C, et al. What population reveals about individual cell identity: Single-cell parameter estimation of models of gene expression in yeast [J]. PLoS computational biology, 2016, 12 (2): e1004706.

[22] MEROUANE A, REY-VILLAMIZAR N, LU Y, et al. Automated profiling of individual cell-cell interactions from high-throughput time-lapse imaging microscopy in nanowell grids (TIMING) [J]. Bioinformatics, 2015, 31 (19): 3189 – 3197.

[23] COMBS C A. Fluorescence microscopy: a concise guide to current imaging methods [J]. Current protocols in neuroscience, 2010 (2): 1

[24] STEPHENS D J, ALLAN V J. Light microscopy techniques for live cell imaging [J]. Science, 2003, 300 (5616): 82 – 86.

[25] CHALFIE M, TU Y, EUSKIRCHEN G, et al. Green fluorescent protein as a marker for gene expression [J]. Science, 1994, 263 (5148): 802 – 805.

[26] SHIMOMURA O, JOHNSON F H, SAIGA Y. Extraction, purification and properties of aequorin, a bioluminescent protein from the luminous hydromedusan, Aequorea [J]. Journal of cellular and comparative physiology, 1962, 59: 223 – 239.

[27] MAGIDSON V, KHODJAKOV A. Circumventing photodamage in live-cell microscopy [J]. Methods in cell biology, 2013, 114: 545 – 560.

[28] WHITE J, STELZER E. Photobleaching GFP reveals protein dynamics inside live cells [J]. Trends in cell biology, 1999, 9 (2): 61 – 65.

[29] MIYAWAKI A. Proteins on the move: insights gained from fluorescent protein technologies [J]. Nature reviews molecular cell biology, 2011, 12 (10): 656 – 668.

[30] KENWORTHY A K. Imaging protein-protein interactions using fluorescence resonance energy transfer microscopy [J]. Methods, 2001, 24 (3): 289 – 296.

[31] PLACHTA N, BOLLENBACH T, PEASE S, et al. Oct4 kinetics predict cell lineage patterning in the early mammalian embryo [J]. Nature cell biology, 2011, 13 (2): 117 – 123.

[32] FIERRO-GONZÁLEZ J C, WHITE M D, SILVA J C, et al. Cadherin-dependent filopodia control preimplantation embryo compaction [J]. Nature cell biology, 2013, 15 (12): 1424-1433.

[33] WHITE M D, ANGIOLINI J F, ALVAREZ Y D, et al. Long-lived binding of Sox2 to DNA predicts cell fate in the four-cell mouse embryo [J]. Cell, 2016, 165 (1): 75-87.

[34] KAUR G, COSTA M W, NEFZGER C M, et al. Probing transcription factor diffusion dynamics in the living mammalian embryo with photoactivatable fluorescence correlation spectroscopy [J]. Nature communications, 2013, 4: 1637.

[35] BOXMAN J, SAGY N, ACHANTA S, et al. Integrated live imaging and molecular profiling of embryoid bodies reveals a synchronized progression of early differentiation [J]. Scientific reports, 2016, 6: 31623.

[36] CHEN J J, ZHANG Z J, LI L, et al. Single-molecule dynamics of enhanceosome assembly in embryonic stem cells [J]. Cell, 2014, 156 (6): 1274-1285.

[37] Embryoscope Time-Lapse System [EB/OL]. [2017-01-17]. http://www.vitrolife.com/sv/Products/EmbryoScope-Time-Lapse-System/.

[38] Primo Vision Time-Lapse System [EB/OL]. [2017-01-17]. http://www.vitrolife.com/en/Fertility/Products/Primo-Vision-Time-Lapse-System/.

[39] Eeva [EB/OL]. [2017-01-17]. https://www.eevatest.com/.

[40] EVANS C L, XIE X S. Coherent anti-stokes Raman scattering microscopy: chemical imaging for biology and medicine [J]. Annual review of analytical chemistry, 2008, 1: 883-909.

[41] TOMER R, KHAIRY K, KELLER P J. Light sheet microscopy in cell biology [J]. Methods in mdecular biology, 2013, 931: 123-137.

[42] PLUTA M. Advanced Light Microscopy (3 Vols.) [M]. New York: Elsevier, 1989.

[43] HOFFMAN R. The modulation contrast microscope: principles and performance [J]. Journal of microscopy, 1977, 110 (3): 205-222.

[44] KOVACS P. Embryo selection: the role of time-lapse monitoring [J]. Reproductive biology and endocrinology: RBE, 2014, 12: 124.

[45] POLANSKI L T, COELHO NETO M A, NASTRI C O, et al. Time-lapse embryo imaging for improving reproductive outcomes: systematic review and meta-analysis [J]. Ultrasound in obstetrics and gynecology, 2014, 44 (4): 394-401.

[46] KAHRAMAN S, ÇETINKAYA M, PIRKEVI C, et al. Comparison of blastocyst development and cycle outcome in patients with eSET using either conventional or time lapse incubators. A prospective study of good prognosis patients [J]. Journal of reproductive and stem cell biotechnology, 2012, 3 (2): 55-61.

[47] KIRKEGAARD K, HINDKJAER J J, GRØNDAHL M L, et al. A randomized clinical trial comparing embryo culture in a conventional incubator with a time-lapse incubator

[J]. Journal of assisted reproduction and genetics, 2012, 29 (6): 565-572.

[48] PARK H, BERGH C, SELLESKOG U, et al. No benefit of culturing embryos in a closed system compared with a conventional incubator in terms of number of good quality embryos: results from an RCT [J]. Human reproduction, 2015, 30 (2): 268-275.

[49] PATERNOT G, WETZELS A M, THONON F, et al. Intra-and inter-observer analysis in the morphological assessment of early stage embryos during an IVF procedure: a multicentre study [J]. Reproductive biology and endocrinology, 2011, 9: 127.

[50] SUNDVALL L, INGERSLEV H J, KNUDSEN U B, et al. Inter-and intra-observer variability of time-lapse annotations [J]. Human reproduction, 2013 (28): 3215-3221.

[51] ALLAN C, BUREL J M, MOORE J, et al. OMERO: flexible, model-driven data management for experimental biology [J]. Nature methods, 2012, 9 (3): 245-253.

[52] BEUCHAT A, THÉVENAZ P, UNSER M, et al. Quantitative morphometrical characterization of human pronuclear zygotes [J]. Human reproduction, 2008, 23 (9): 1983-1992.

[53] FILHO E S, NOBLE J A, WELLS D. A review on automatic analysis of human embryo microscope images [J]. The open biomedical engineering journal, 2010, 4: 170-177.

[54] GIUSTI A, CORANI G, GAMBARDELLA L M, et al. Blastomere segmentation and 3D morphology measurements of early embryos from Hoffman Modulation Contrast image stacks [C]//IEEE International Symposium on Biomedical Imaging. Rotterdam, Netherlands: IEEE, 2010: 1261-1264.

[55] WONG C C, LOEWKE K E, BOSSERT N L, et al. Non-invasive imaging of human embryos before embryonic genome activation predicts development to the blastocyst stage [J]. Nature biotechnology, 2010, 28 (10): 1115-1121.

[56] MOUSSAVI F, WANG Y, LORENZEN P, et al. A unified graphical models framework for automated mitosis detection in human embryos [J]. IEEE transactions on medical imaging, 2014, 33 (7): 1551-1562.

[57] AGERHOLM I E, HNIDA C, CRUGER D G, et al. Nuclei size in relation to nuclear status and aneuploidy rate for 13 chromosomes in donated four cells embryos [J]. Journal of assisted reproduction and genetics, 2008, 25 (2-3): 95-102.

[58] MORALES D A, BENGOETXEA E, LARRANAGA P. Automatic segmentation of zona pellucida in human embryo images applying an active contour model [J]. Proc 12th Annu Conf Med Image Underst Anal, 2008, 209-213.

[59] FILHO E S, NOBLE J A, POLI M, et al. A method for semi-automatic grading of human blastocyst microscope images [J]. Human reproduction, 2012, 27 (9): 2641-2648.

[60] KANG M J, XENOPOULOS P, MUÑOZ-DESCALZO S, et al. Live imaging, identifying, and tracking single cells in complex populations in vivo and ex vivo [J]. Methods in molecular biology, 2013, 1052: 109-123.

[61] TURKSEN K. Imaging and tracking stem cells: methods and protocols [M]. New York, USA: New York Humana Press, 2013.

[62] TSIEN R Y. The green fluorescent protein [J]. Annual review of biochemistry, 1998, 67: 509-544.

[63] FINE A. Confocal microscopy: principles and practice. Chapter 6, Yuste R & Konnerth A editors. In Imaging in Neuroscience and Development [M]. New York, USA: Cold Spring Harbor Laboratory Press, Cold Spring Harbor; 2005.

[64] USTIONE A, PISTON D W. A simple introduction to multiphoton microscopy [J]. Journal of microscopy, 2011, 243 (3): 221-226.

[65] SAMARAGE C R, WHITE M D, ÁLVAREZ Y D, et al. Cortical tension allocates the first inner cells of the mammalian embryo [J]. Developmental cell, 2015, 34 (4): 435-447.

[66] TURNER D L, WEINTRAUB H. Expression of achaete-scute homolog 3 in Xenopus embryos converts ectodermal cells to a neural fate [J]. Genes and development, 1994, 8 (12): 1434-1447.

[67] LOUVET-VALLÉE S, DARD N, SANTA-MARIA A, et al. A major posttranslational modification of ezrin takes place during epithelial differentiation in the early mouse embryo [J]. Developments in biologicals, 2001, 231 (1): 190-200.

[68] KHAN A, GOULD S, SALZMANN M. Segmentation of developing human embryo in time-lapse microscopy [C]//IEEE International Symposium on Biomedical Imaging. Prague, Czech Republic: IEEE, 2016: 930-934.

[69] KHAN A, GOULD S, SALZMANN M. Automated monitoring of human embryonic cells up to the 5-cell stage in time-lapse microscopy images [C]//12th IEEE International Symposium on Biomedical Imaging. NY USA: IEEE, 2015: 389-393.

[70] KHAN A, GOULD S, SALZMANN M. A linear chain Markov model for detection and localization of cells in early stage embryo development [C]//IEEE Winter Conference on Applications of Computer Vision. Waikoloa, HI, USA: IEEE, 2015, 526-533.

[71] KHAN A, GOULD S, SALZMANN M. Deep convolutional neural networks for human embryonic cell counting [C]//Workshop on Bioimage Computing at European Conference on Computer Vision (ECCV). Amsterdam, Netherlands: Springer, 2016, 339-348.

[72] KHAN A, GOULD S, SALZMANN M. Detecting abnormal cell division patterns in early-stage human embryo development [C]//Machine Learning in Medical Imaging (MLMI). Munich, Germany: Springer, 2015, 161-169.

[73] MÖLDER A, DRURY S, COSTEN N, et al. Semiautomated analysis of embryoscope images: Using localized variance of image intensity to detect embryo developmental stages [J]. Cytometry. Part A: 2015, 87 (2): 119-128.

[74] MÖLDER A, CZANNER S, COSTEN N, et al. Automatic detection of circular structures in human embryo imaging using trigonometric rotation of the Hough Transform.

［C］//IEEE 22nd International Conference on Pattern Recognition (ICPR). Stockholm, Sweden: IEEE, 2014, 3239-3244.

［75］DEGLINCERTI A, CROFT G F, PIETILA L N, et al. Self-organization of the in vitro attached human embryo［J］. Nature, 2016, 533 (7602): 251-254.

［76］MÖLDER A, CZANNER S, COSTEN N. Focal plane selection in microscopic embryo images［C］//TPCG Conference on Computer Graphics & Visual Computing. Leeds, United Kingdom: TPCG, 2014: 29-31.

(Anna Leida Mölder, Juan Carlos Fierro-González and Aisha Khan)

第5章　胚胎基因表达和表观遗传学的控制

> 着床前胚胎发育遵循一系列关键事件：显著的表观遗传修饰和基因表达重编程出现能够启动胚胎基因组。在植入前胚胎发育早期阶段，母体 mRNAs 指导着胚胎发育。在整个早期胚胎发育过程中，尽管部分阶段表现出特异性变化，但主要维持着不同的甲基化模式。最近的研究表明，不同的去甲基化过程引起早期发育胚胎中不同的亲本基因差异表达，这可能会影响胚胎的正确发育。近年来，非编码 RNA、长链非编码 RNA（lncRNA）和短链 miRNA 在胚胎着床前发育中的作用越来越受到重视。

着床前胚胎发育遵循一系列关键事件。这些事件始于配子发生、成熟配子的形成，一直持续到分娩结束。雄性和雌性配子分别从原始生殖细胞（primordial germ cells，PGCs）中分化而来，通过精子发生和卵子发生过程得以获得。PGCs 具有独特的基因表达、表观遗传学、形态学和行为学特性。PGCs 一旦经历有丝分裂，在不同性别间精子发生和卵子发生的进展就表现出差异。在精子发生过程中，精原细胞从青春期开始进行有丝分裂直到死亡为止，每个初级精母细胞在减数分裂结束时可产生 4 个精子细胞。在卵子发生过程中，PGCs 分化为卵原细胞，进入减数分裂并停止分化，直至青春期重新启动。与精子发生中的第二次减数分裂不同，卵母细胞在受精之前不会完成第二次减数分裂。随着第二次减数分裂的完成，每个卵原细胞仅可产生 1 个存活的卵母细胞[1]。

受精时，卵母细胞完成减数分裂，完成受精的卵母细胞称为合子，即卵母细胞和精子核融合形成合子（图 5-1）。合子经历一系列分裂，形成两细胞、四细胞、八细胞、桑葚胚和囊胚[2]（图 5-1）。在胚胎分裂早期，母系和父系的染色体发生程序性变性以激活胚胎基因组（又称胚胎基因组激活，embryonic genome activation，EGA），并启动着床前胚胎发育。如果 EGA 失败，胚胎基因组未启动则胚胎无法发挥细胞分裂功能，胚胎发育就会停止[3]。这是由母体核酸、储存在卵母细胞中的特异性 RNA、蛋白质和其他大分子降解启动的[4]。EGA 开始于小鼠的两细胞期，在人类则是四细胞期至八细胞期[5]，在植入前胚胎中发生了显著的重编程表达。这些重编程事件由 DNA 甲基化、组蛋白乙酰化、转录、翻译和 miRNA 调节等共同调控[6]。因此，着床前胚胎的发育包括连续的分子、细胞和形态学变迁事件。这些事件最终将形成一个多维度胚胎，具有着床和继续发育的潜能。

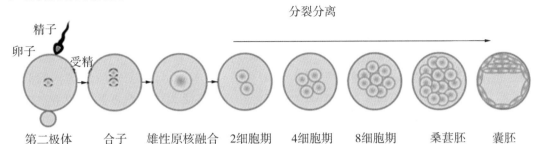

受精后的合子，胚胎分裂产生2个、3个、4个等细胞胚胎，最终形成桑葚胚和囊胚。

图5-1 植入前胚胎发育主要阶段示意

本章将讨论在植入前胚胎发育过程中影响基因表达的不同因子。将对配子和着床前胚胎的表观遗传因子（侧重于甲基化谱）进行综述。非编码 RNA 对基因表达的影响也将在本章中做出评估。

1 基因表达与表观遗传学

对于正常发育的胚胎，需要母系基因和父系基因均正常表达。受精后发生强烈的表观遗传变化，才能建立早期胚胎的多能性[7]。染色质存在许多翻译后修饰（主要包括乙酰化、泛素化、苏酰化和磷酸化），其中，组蛋白赖氨酸和精氨酸残基的甲基化修饰是植入前胚胎的表观遗传学变化的焦点。

DNA 甲基化和染色质修饰不仅在决定转录状态中起着关键作用，而且能够决定转录抑制[8-10]。导致甲基化变化的机制尚未完全确定，但有人认为重编程是通过被动或主动去甲基化完成的。去甲基化与 DNA 修复有关[11-14]。DNA 甲基化主要在 PGC 形成和着床前胚胎两阶段的发育中起着重要调控作用。

1.1 合子和着床前胚胎的表观遗传修饰

在哺乳动物（人、牛、大鼠、猪和小鼠）胚胎发育中，除印记基因外，受精卵全基因组均经历一次去甲基化过程[15-18]。由于 DNA 复制的丢失，导致姐妹染色单体出现不对称甲基化状态，合子中的雄性原核经历选择性去甲基化过程[15-16,19-20]。这些事件是在人类和小鼠精子受精后解聚开始时发生的[17,21-22]。在此阶段，合子的雌性原核仍然高度甲基化[17,21-22]。母体基因组的去甲基化始于胚胎第一次分裂[19,23-24]。到桑葚胚阶段，小鼠的植入前胚胎甲基化不足。大约在发育中胚胎的八细胞期出现单个卵裂球的极化和致密化。这些过程涉及许多调节因子，包括 E-钙黏蛋白（CDH1）、分配缺陷同系物 3（PARD3）、分配缺陷同系物 6B（PARD6B）和蛋白激酶 C zeta[25-27]。

囊胚期胚胎由 1 个充满液体的空腔和由内细胞团（ICM）和滋养外胚层（TE）组

成的细胞群组成。胚胎发育到四细胞期至八细胞期，这些细胞可同时形成 ICM 和 TE 的完整谱系，所有卵裂球被认为具有全能性[28]。ICM 发育成胎儿，而 TE 形成胚胎外组织，如胎盘。ICM 由多能干细胞组成，这些细胞有能力发育成胎儿的任何细胞类型。转录和表观遗传事件严格控制这些分化事件。许多转录因子在囊胚形成中起着关键作用，其中包括用于 TE 形成的尾侧同源框 2（CDX2）、用于建立 ICM 多能性的八聚体 3（OCT3）/八聚体 4（OCT4）和 NANOG[29-31]。CDX2 广泛表达于八细胞期和十六细胞期，而在囊胚中仅在 TE 细胞中表达[32]。尽管 OCT4 和 NANOG 也广泛表达于八细胞期和十六细胞期胚胎，但它们仅在囊胚的 ICM 中表达[32]。囊胚的形成需要许多转录因子。缺乏 CDX2 表达的胚胎不能形成囊胚腔，但它们具有着床潜能[30]。缺乏 OCT4 或 NANOG 表达的胚胎会导致 ICM 形成失败，这些胚胎的囊胚发育会受阻[31-32]。TEAD4 是另一种在囊胚形成中起作用的转录因子，TEAD4 核定位的缺失会损害囊胚中 TE 特异性转录程序[33]。此外，TCFAP2C 转录因子的异常表达也会导致桑葚胚到囊胚过渡期间的胚胎停滞[34]，Klf5 小鼠突变胚胎会停滞在囊胚阶段[35]。

DNA 重新甲基化过程在胚胎植入后不久开始发生[16, 22-23, 36]。这种从头甲基化不对称发生，因此 ICM 可能由于 Dnmt3b 甲基化酶高表达而出现高度甲基化[37]，而 TE 由于酶催化的主动去甲基化和被动去甲基化而保持低甲基化[11, 14, 22]。胚胎中甲基化谱的改变已被证明会导致 ICM 和 TE 分化的改变。H3 精氨酸 26 残基甲基化（H3R26me）的变化也参与卵裂球 TE 和 ICM 分化的变化[38]。

X 染色体失活也是一种表观遗传学现象，其中 X 染色体的活性受到严格的调控，以平衡男性和女性之间以及相对于常染色体的 X 染色体表达和基因剂量的差异[39]。正常的发育过程中，X 染色体剂量补偿至关重要。X 染色体的失活至少发生在 2 个阶段：失活的起始和维持。X 染色体失活小鼠模型系统表明，X 染色体失活发生在早期胚胎发育期间，通过 X 染色体上基因的转录沉默而失活[40]。研究表明，在人类植入前胚胎中女性 X 染色体表达的减少保障了剂量补偿[41]。LncRNA-XIST 表达通过参与染色质重塑的蛋白质启动 X 染色体失活[3, 42]。单细胞 RNA 测序技术证实了 lncRNAs XACT 和在早期人类植入前胚胎的活性可影响 X 染色体表达[43]。此外，这两种 RNA 的表达从未显示出重叠。将 XACT 导入异源系统导致 XIST-RNA 在 cis 中的积累，它可能参与控制 XIST 与 cis 染色体的关联，并可能调节其沉默能力。XACT 也可能在着床前胚胎发育的早期阶段平衡 X 染色体失活[43-44]。最近，剂量补偿被证明是由一个新的 XIST 等位基因［XIST（CAG）］的 CAG 启动子驱动的[45]。此外，着床前胚胎中的 XIST（CAG）上调表现出依赖于亲本来源的变化，并且父系表达建议优先通过父系 XIST（CAG）传播失活[45]。

1.2 配子的表观遗传修饰

在生殖细胞中，甲基化以性别特异的方式维持。PGCs 的甲基化水平随着它们迁移到性腺而减少。研究表明，雌性的卵母细胞在出生后持续发育而发生再甲基化过程。雄性 PGCs 进入有丝分裂或雌性 PGCs 在减数分裂停止时，去甲基化完成[46]。

胚胎中甲基化的重新编程对于基因的亲本特异性表达是必须的[14]。由于这些重编程事件，基因表达在植入前胚胎发育过程中发生变化，适当的基因表达决定了胚胎的存活[6]。最近，短链非编码 RNA、miRNAs 和长链非编码 RNA（lncRNA）在其潜在功能中变得非常重要，它们可以通过靶向多个基因影响多种生理生化途径[47-48]。

2 基因表达和短链非编码 RNA：miRNA

miRNA 是一个长度为 17～25 个核苷酸（nt）的短链非编码 RNA 大家族[49]。20 多年前，在秀丽隐杆线虫中首次发现了 miRNA[50]，此后，通过分子克隆和生物信息学技术，许多 miRNA 已在多种生物体中被发现，如蠕虫、苍蝇、鱼、青蛙、哺乳动物和植物[51]。大多数 miRNA 序列在许多哺乳动物中都是保守的[52]，尽管有些 miRNA 序列彼此之间存在一个核苷酸的差异[53]。不同物种之间的保守 miRNA 序列可以通过命名法来区分。因此，当 miRNA 序列中只有前 3 个字母不同时，表明为不同物种中的相同序列，如智人中的 hsa-miR-145 和小家鼠中的 mmu-miR-145[54]。

miRNAs 在涉及细胞周期调节、凋亡、细胞分化、印迹基因、内环境稳定和发育等多种生物学过程中扮演重要作用，还包括肢体发育[55]、肺上皮的形态发生[56]、胚胎血管生成[57]、毛囊的形成和 T 细胞的增殖[58-59]。miRNAs 通过靶向 mRNAs 进行翻译抑制、切割、降解或失稳，在调节许多生物体的转录和转录后基因沉默中发挥关键作用[53, 60-64]。每个 miRNA 都有多个 mRNA 靶点，可调节高达 30% 的蛋白质编码基因，并影响数百到数千个基因的蛋白质生产[65-67]。miRNA 通过在靶 mRNA 的开放阅读框（open reading frame，ORF）和 3′非翻译区（3′untranslated region，UTR）内的种子序列互补序列（2-8nT 的 miRNA）的碱基配对来识别其靶基因[68]。尽管 miRNAs 的靶点尚不完全清楚，但生物信息学研究显示了一系列可能的靶基因[69]。利用 miRNA 数据库可以识别 miRNA 的功能活性和预测/观察到的靶点。（可以使用以下网址访问这些数据库：http：// www. targetscan. org/；http：//www. microrna. org/microrna/home. do；http：//mirdb. org/miRDB/。）

2.1 miRNA 生物发生

miRNA 生物发生涉及多个重要步骤。miRNA 首先通过 RNA 聚合酶 II 从基因组 DNA 转录到初级 miRNA（pri-miRNA），初级 miRNA 含有茎环结构。Drosha 是一种相对分子量为 30～160 kDa 的蛋白质酶，具有 1 个双链 RNA 结合域和 2 个催化域[70]。在 DGCR8 存在的情况下，对发夹的 2 条链进行切割，产生约 70 nt 大小的前 miRNA 产物（pre-miRNA）[71]。这些前 miRNA 通过 Exportin-5（Exp5）从细胞核进入细胞质，Exportin-5 是核质转运蛋白家族中的一种核质转运蛋白，存在 RAs 相关核蛋白（Ran）和鸟苷三磷酸（guanosine triphosphate，GTP）的情况下，具有前 miRNA 的结合位点[72-73]。这些 miRNA 被细胞质核糖核酸酶内切酶 Dicer 进一步切割，形成 21～22 nt 双链结构。其中 1 条链通常被降解，前 miRNA 的 2 条链可能与含 Argonaute（Ago）蛋白的复合物相关，

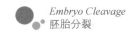

并且它们由 RISC/miRNP（RNA 诱导沉默复合物/mi‐核糖核蛋白）介导形成单链成熟 miRNA。与 RISC 相关的 miRNA 主要针对靶标 mRNA，它们要么抑制其翻译，要么使 mRNA 降解，导致蛋白质合成减少[70, 74]。

研究表明，Dicer 酶对 miRNA 的形成至关重要，任何 *Dicer* 缺陷（如发育中动物的 *Dicer* 的缺失）都会导致动物畸变[75-76]。果蝇生殖系干细胞缺乏 *Dicer* 延缓了 G1/S 期转换[77]，这表明 miRNA 可能是干细胞发育绕过该关键点的关键。在小鼠和秀丽隐杆线虫的 *Dicer* 突变中，分别观察到卵母细胞纺锤体减少和紊乱、染色体排列错误以及原肠胚形成缺陷[50, 78]。在斑马鱼和秀丽隐杆线虫体内注射 miR-430 可部分修复原肠胚形成、视网膜发育和生长发育[78]。斑马鱼、小鼠和海马中的 *Dicer* 缺失导致神经系统出现问题，并导致无法形成成熟的 miRNA，从而导致大脑形态发生和神经元分化的变化[79-80]。母体‐合子 *Dicer* 的突变，斑马鱼和小鼠胚胎的轴形成和早期分化是正常的，但仍然引发了体细胞发生、形态发生方面的缺陷，分别影响大脑形成、原肠胚形成、心脏发育和肢体中胚层的凋亡[78, 81-83]。*Dicer*-null 小鼠发育的肢体中胚层细胞凋亡增强[84]。Dicer 缺陷会导致第 7.5 天左右的小鼠胚胎死亡[50, 78, 85]和早期斑马鱼胚胎死亡[86]，这体现了 miRNA 介导的基因沉默在母体到合子转变中的重要性。

小鼠生殖道体细胞中 *Dicer*1 的完全缺失不仅导致 miRNA 的表达量减少，而且还导致雌性小鼠不育，卵母细胞和胚胎完整性受损[50, 87]。*Dicer* 缺陷雄性小鼠的精原细胞增殖特性不良。雄性小鼠生殖系（纯合子 Dicer1）中 *Dicer*1 的缺失导致精子发生异常，生育能力下降，生殖细胞数量减少，精子细胞异常，精母细胞表型异常，核浓缩，精子活力异常，睾丸支持小管突变[88]。研究表明，母体细胞质 *Dicer* 的转移掩盖了早期异常表型[78-89]。

敲除小鼠胚胎成纤维细胞和造血细胞中的 *Ago*2 导致成熟 miRNA 表达水平降低[61, 90-91]。研究发现，*Ago*2 缺陷卵母细胞发育过程中出现具有异常纺锤体的成熟卵母细胞，染色体不能正常结合，miRNA 表达水平降低（超过 80%）。*Ago*2 功能丧失导致小鼠在胚胎第 9.5 天左右死亡[92]。

2.2　miRNA 在着床前胚胎中的表达

植入前胚胎中 miRNA 的表达主要通过敲除实验、克隆实验以及微阵列分析和反转录聚合酶链反应（reverse transcription PCR，RT-PCR）鉴定单个 miRNA 进行研究[93]。人们使用动物模型、组织、培养细胞进行了 miRNA 表达研究；也可以在癌细胞、人类胚胎干细胞，以及小鼠、牛或人的配子和胚胎中进行了广泛的研究。人类胚胎干细胞来源于囊胚期的内细胞团，具有自我更新和多向分化的能力；人类胚胎相关材料的获取非常困难，人类胚胎干细胞是研究相关基因表达的关键材料，也是最接近人类胚胎的代表之一。研究人类胚胎干细胞中 miRNA 的表达，不仅可以深入了解人类胚胎中潜在 miR-NA 的表达情况，还可以研究 miRNA 在干细胞功能中发挥的重要作用[94]。

在小鼠、牛和人类的卵子发生和精子发生过程中就已观察到了 miRNA 的表达[95-96]。在未成熟卵母细胞和成熟卵母细胞观察到 miRNA 的差异表达，这可能代表自然更新的状态，也表明每个胚胎阶段由特定的 miRNA 表达差异所影响。成熟小鼠卵母细胞和早期发育胚胎中类似的 miRNA 表达谱表明，在上述阶段合子具有母体遗传的 miRNA[50]。与卵母细胞类似，精子也携带一系列 miRNA。大约 20% 的 miRNA 位于精子的细胞核或核周部分，表明这些 miRNA 在受精时可转移到受精卵中[97]。有人认为，精子携带的 miRNA 可能下调哺乳动物的母体转录本；然而，使用微阵列分析对这一假设进行检验时，发现精子中的这些 miRNA 均不具有重要意义，因为它们的相同序列都已经存在于卵母细胞中（减数分裂Ⅱ）[98]。

多个 miRNA 参与生殖细胞层的形成。在小鼠胚胎着床前，胚胎发育过程中不同表达水平的 miR-290 通过靶向淋巴结抑制小鼠胚胎干细胞中的生殖细胞和中胚层分化产生负面调节[99]。在斑马鱼中，miR-290 簇在调节中胚层诱导中发挥了正向作用[100]。因此，尚不清楚 miR-290 对中胚层分化是否有抑制作用。其他 miRNA（如 miR-15 和 miR-16[100]）已被证明对斑马鱼中胚层分化有影响，这些 miRNAs 也在小鼠植入前胚胎中存在表达[50]。

在小鼠和牛胚胎的卵裂过程中表达相同的 miRNA。然而，它们的表达水平往往存在差异。例如在小鼠胚胎中，miRNA 表达水平在一细胞期和二细胞期之间降低多达 60%。在四细胞期结束时，小鼠胚胎的 miRNA 含量大约是二细胞期胚胎的 2 倍。这意味着母系遗传的 miRNA 在此阶段降解，EGA 开始于单细胞期至四细胞期[50]。在小鼠着床前胚胎发育过程中，miRNA 的合成和降解共存，但在囊胚期总体 miRNA 表达增加[101]。

在人类中已经鉴定出 700 多个 miRNA[87, 95-96, 102]。在卵母细胞和囊胚阶段，大多数 miRNA 的表达水平保持不变[87]。另外，人类卵母细胞和囊胚中表达的 miRNA 中有 50% 以上与肿瘤发生有关，如 let-7 家族、miR-19a、miR-21 和 miR-34[103-109]。

3　基因表达与长链非编码 RNA

在过去的几年中，除了短链非编码 RNA 外，长链非编码 RNA（lncRNA）在影响基因表达中的作用也越来越得到重视。哺乳动物基因组的长基因间非编码 RNA（lincRNA）在着床前胚胎发育过程中发挥多能性调节作用[110]。据报道，人类多能性转录本 2、3 和 5（HPAT2、HPAT3 和 HPAT5）可调节着床前胚胎的多能性和 ICM 形成。此外，HPAT5 被证明与 let-7 miRNA 家族相互作用[110]。

胚胎移植涉及复杂的机制，移植过程中涉及许多不同的遗传和生理因素。发育中的着床前胚胎必须与母体子宫内膜有良好的协同作用。动物研究显示，lncRNA 在妊娠猪和非妊娠猪的子宫内膜组织中显示出差异表达，两种 lncRNA（TCONS_01729386 和 TCONS_01325501）在着床中具有潜在作用[111]。

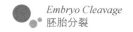

4 基因表达与人类辅助生殖技术

在西方国家，大约1%的儿童是通过辅助生殖技术（ART）出生的。不孕夫妇通过该技术获得最大的怀孕可能。尽管 ART 在胎儿发育和产后发育方面被认为是安全可靠的[112-113]，但也有报道显示通过 ART 生育的孩子患病风险增加，尤其是印记基因障碍相关的疾病有增加[114]。此外，由于合子的体外培养[115-116]和体外受精过程[117]，基因表达谱也有所不同。体外培养后，胚胎凋亡和形态发生途径与正常体内发育胚胎显示出差异变化[118]。

卵胞质内单精子注射（ICSI）是广泛使用的 ART 之一，它为精子活力有问题的不孕夫妇提供了生孩子的绝好机会。ICSI 是一个独特的过程，在这个过程中，单个被挑选的精子被注入卵子胞浆中[119]。然而，ICSI 绕过了一些正常受精过程中发生的生理过程。这些来自 ICSI 的胚胎被证明以较慢的速度分裂，且胚胎孵化数量减少，细胞数量减少，钙振荡缩短，与正常胚胎发育模式不同[120]。ICSI 产生的小鼠胚胎被证明有肥胖趋势并伴有器官发育异常[121]。

5 结论

植入前胚胎的正常发育涉及极其复杂的机制。对于正常发育的胚胎，需要母系和父系基因正常的表达。在着床前胚胎中，亲本基因的调控涉及多种因素。表观遗传修饰是影响着床前胚胎基因表达调控的重要因素之一。多年来，为了建立哺乳动物配子和胚胎的甲基化谱，人们进行了广泛的研究。近几年来，非编码 RNA 在基因调控中的作用变得越来越明显。目前已进行了一些研究分析 miRNA 的表达，表明 miRNA 可以调节编码高达 30% 人类蛋白质编码基因的 mRNAs。在小鼠、牛和人的配子和胚胎中也观察到了 miRNA 的表达和功能调节。此外，长链非编码 RNA 的表达及其在胚胎发育和着床中的作用已被广泛研究。广泛的研究为着床前胚胎的发育和基因表达的调控提供了重要的途径，随着技术的进步，更多的分子相关研究将有助于更好地理解其机制。

参考文献

[1] JAROUDI S, SENGUPTA S. DNA repair in mammalian embryos [J]. Mutation research, 2007, 635（1）：53-77.

[2] WILLIAM L. Human embryology [M]. 2nd ed. New York：Churchill Livingstone,

1997.

[3] SCHULTZ RM. The molecular foundations of the maternal to zygotic transition in the pre-implantation embryo [J]. Human reproduction update, 2002, 8 (4): 323-331.

[4] MOORE K, PERSAUD TVN. The Developing Human [M]. 6th ed. Philadelphia: Saunders Company, 1998.

[5] TELFORD N A, WATSON A J, SCHULTZ G A. Transition from maternal to embryonic control in early mammalian development: a comparison of several species [J]. Molecular reproduction and development, 1990, 26 (1): 90-100.

[6] BELL C E, CALDER M D, WATSON A J. Genomic RNA profiling and the programme controlling preimplantation mammalian development [J]. Molecular human reproduction, 2008, 14 (12): 691-701.

[7] MCCLAY D W, CLARKE H J. Remodelling the paternal chromatin at fertilisation in mammals [J]. Reproduction, 2003, 125 (5): 625-633.

[8] TAMARU H, SELKER E U. A histone H3 methyltransferase controls DNA methylation in *Neurospora crassa* [J]. Nature, 2001, 414 (6861): 277-283.

[9] JACKSON J P, LINDROTH A M, CAO X, et al. Control of CpNpG DNA methylation by the KRYPTONITE histone H3 methyltransferase [J]. Nature, 2002, 416 (6880): 556-560.

[10] FUKS F, HURD P J, WOLF D, et al. The methyl-CpG-binding protein MeCP2 links DNA methylation to histone methylation [J]. The journal of biological chemistry, 2003, 278 (6): 4035-4040.

[11] MORGAN H D, SANTOS F, GREEN K, et al. Epigenetic reprogramming in mammals [J]. Human molecular genetics, 2005, 14 (Spec No 1): R47-R58.

[12] ZHU B, ZHENG Y, ANGLIKER H, et al. 5-Methylcytosine DNA glycosylase activity is also present in the human MBD4 (G/T mismatch glycosylase) and in a related avian sequence [J]. Nucleic acids research, 2000, 28 (21): 4157-4165.

[13] HARDELAND U, BENTELE M, JIRICNY J, et al. The versatile thymine DNA-glycosylase: a comparative characterization of the human, Drosophila and fission yeast orthologs [J]. Nucleic acids research, 2003, 31 (9): 2261-2271.

[14] DEAN W, LUCIFERO D, SANTOS F. DNA methylation in mammalian development and disease [J]. Birth defects research. Part C, embryo today: reviews, 2005, 75 (2): 98-111.

[15] OSWALD J, ENGEMANN S, LANE N, et al. Active demethylation of the paternal genome in the mouse zygote [J]. Current biology, 2000, 10 (8): 475-478.

[16] MAYER W, NIVELEAU A, WALTER J, et al. Demethylation of the zygotic paternal genome [J]. Nature, 2000, 403 (6769): 501-502.

[17] BEAUJEAN N, HARTSHORNE G, CAVILLA J, et al. Non-conservation of mammalian preimplantation methylation dynamics [J]. Current biology, 2004, 14 (7): R266-

R267.

[18] REIK W, DEAN W, WALTER J. Epigenetic reprogramming in mammalian development [J]. Science, 2001, 293 (1089): 1089 – 1093.

[19] ROUGIER N, BOURC'HIS D, GOMES D M, et al. Chromosome methylation patterns during mammalian preimplantation development [J]. Genes & development, 1998, 12 (14): 2108 – 2113.

[20] DEAN W, SANTOS F, STOJKOVIC M, et al. Conservation of methylation reprogramming in mammalian development: aberrant reprogramming in cloned embryos [J]. Proceedings of the National Academy of Sciences of the United States of America, 2001, 98 (24): 13734 – 13738.

[21] SANTOS F, DEAN W. Epigenetic reprogramming during early development in mammals [J]. Reproduction, 2004, 127 (6): 643 – 651.

[22] SANTOS F, HENDRICH B, REIK W, et al. Dynamic reprogramming of DNA methylation in the early mouse embryo [J]. Developmental biology, 2002, 241 (1): 172 – 182.

[23] MONK M, BOUBELIK M, LEHNERT S. Temporal and regional changes in DNA methylation in the embryonic, extraembryonic and germ cell lineages during mouse embryo development [J]. Development, 1987, 99 (3): 371 – 382.

[24] HOWLETT S K, REIK W. Methylation levels of maternal and paternal genomes during preimplantation development [J]. Development, 1991, 113 (1): 119 – 127.

[25] DE VRIES W N, EVSIKOV A V, HAAC B E, et al. Maternal beta-catenin and E-cadherin in mouse development [J]. Development, 2004, 131 (18): 4435 – 4445.

[26] ALARCON V B. Cell polarity regulator PARD6B is essential for trophectoderm formation in the preimplantation mouse embryo [J]. Biology of reproduction, 2010, 83 (3): 347 – 358.

[27] DUCIBELLA T, UKENA T, KARNOVSKY M, et al. Changes in cell surface and cortical cytoplasmic organization during early embryogenesis in the preimplantation mouse embryo [J]. The journal of biological chemistry, 1977, 74 (1): 153 – 167.

[28] KELLY S J, Studies of the developmental potential of 4-and 8-cell stage mouse blastomeres [J]. The journal of experimental zoology, 1977, 200 (3): 365 – 376.

[29] CHAMBERS I, COLBY D, ROBERTSON M, et al. Functional expression cloning of Nanog, a pluripotency sustaining factor in embryonic stem cells [J]. Cell, 2003, 113 (5): 643 – 655.

[30] STRUMPF D, MAO C A, YAMANAKA Y, et al. Cdx2 is required for correct cell fate specification and differentiation of trophectoderm in the mouse blastocyst [J]. Development, 2005, 132 (9): 2093 – 2102.

[31] NICHOLS J, ZEVNIK B, ANASTASSIADIS K, et al. Formation of pluripotent stem cells in the mammalian embryo depends on the POU transcription factor Oct4 [J]. Cell,

1998, 95 (3): 379-391.

[32] DIETRICH J E, HIIRAGI T. Stochastic patterning in the mouse pre-implantation embryo [J]. Development, 2007, 134 (23): 4219-4231.

[33] HOME P, SAHA B, RAY S, et al. Altered subcellular localization of transcription factor TEAD4 regulates first mammalian cell lineage commitment [J]. Proceedings of the National Academy of Sciences of the United States of America, 2012, 109 (19): 7362-7367.

[34] PAUL S, KNOTT J G. Epigenetic control of cell fate in mouse blastocysts: the role of covalent histone modifications and chromatin remodeling [J]. Molecular reproduction and development, 2014, 81 (2): 171-182.

[35] LIN S C, WANI M A, WHITSETT J A, et al. Klf5 regulates lineage formation in the pre-implantation mouse embryo [J]. Development, 2010, 137 (23): 3953-3963.

[36] DAVIS T L, YANG G J, MCCARREY J R, et al. The H19 methylation imprint is erased and re-established differentially on the parental alleles during male germ cell development [J]. Human molecular genetics, 2000, 9 (19): 2885-2294.

[37] WATANABE D, SUETAKE I, TADA T, et al. Stage-and cell-specific expression of Dnmt3a and Dnmt3b during embryogenesis [J]. Mechanisms of development, 2002, 118 (1-2): 187-190.

[38] TORRES-PADILLA M E, PARFITT D E, KOUZARIDES T, et al. Histone arginine methylation regulates pluripotency in the early mouse embryo [J]. Nature, 2007, 445 (7124): 214-218.

[39] DISTECHE C M. Dosage compensation of the sex chromosomes and autosomes [J]. Seminars in cell & developmental biology semin, 2016, 56: 9-18.

[40] NAMEKAWA S H, PAYER B, HUYNH K D, et al. Two-step imprinted X inactivation: repeat versus genic silencing in the mouse [J]. Molecular and cellular biology, 2010, 30 (13): 3187-3205.

[41] PETROPOULOS S, EDSGÄRD D, REINIUS B, et al. Single-cell RNA-seq reveals lineage and X chromosome dynamics in human preimplantation embryos [J]. Cell, 2016, 165 (4): 1012-1026.

[42] MCHUGH C A, CHEN C K, CHOW A, et al. The Xist lncRNA interacts directly with SHARP to silence transcription through HDAC3 [J]. Nature, 2015, 521 (7551): 232-236.

[43] VALLOT C, PATRAT C, COLLIER A J, et al. XACT noncoding RNA competes with XIST in the control of X chromosome activity during human early development [J]. Cell stem cell, 2017, 20 (1): 102-111.

[44] PETROPOULOS S, EDSGÄRD D, REINIUS B, et al. Single-cell RNA-seq reveals lineage and X chromosome dynamics in human preimplantation embryos [J]. Cell, 2016, 165 (4): 1012-1026.

[45] AMAKAWA Y, SAKATA Y, HOKI Y, et al. A new Xist allele driven by a constitutively active promoter is dominated by Xist locus environment and exhibits the parent-of-origin effects [J]. Development, 2015, 142 (24): 4299-4308.

[46] SEKI Y, HAYASHI K, ITOH K, et al. Extensive and orderly reprogramming of genome-wide chromatin modifications associated with specification and early development of germ cells in mice [J]. Developmental biology, 2005, 278 (2): 440-458.

[47] PLACE R F, LI L C, POOKOT D, et al. MicroRNA-373 induces expression of genes with complementary promoter sequences [J]. Proceedings of the National Academy of Sciences of the United States of America, 2008, 105 (5): 1608-1613.

[48] PLASTERK R H. Micro RNAs in animal development [J]. Cell, 2006, 124 (5): 877-881.

[49] TANG F, KANEDA M, O'CARROLL D, et al. Maternal microRNAs are essential for mouse zygotic development [J]. Genes & development, 2007, 21 (6): 644-648.

[50] LEE R C, FEINBAUM R L, AMBROS V. The *C. elegans* heterochronic gene *lin-4* encodes small RNAs with antisense complementarity to *lin-14* [J]. Cell, 1993, 75 (5): 843-854.

[51] LEE R C, AMBROS V. An extensive class of small RNAs in *Caenorhabditis elegans* [J]. Science, 2001, 294 (5543): 862-864.

[52] NIWA R, SLACK F J. The evolution of animal microRNA function [J]. Current opinion in genetics & development, 2007, 17 (2): 145-150.

[53] TESFAYE D, WORKU D, RINGS F, et al. Identification and expression profiling of microRNAs during bovine oocyte maturation using heterologous approach [J]. Molecular reproduction and development, 2009, 76 (7): 665-677.

[54] GRIFFITHS-JONES S, GROCOCK R J, VAN DONGEN S, et al. miRBase: microRNA sequences, targets and gene nomenclature [J]. Nucleic acids research, 2006, 34 (Database issue): D140-D144.

[55] HARFE B D, MCMANUS M T, MANSFIELD J H, et al. The RNaseIII enzyme *Dicer* is required for morphogenesis but not patterning of the vertebrate limb [J]. Proceedings of the National Academy of Sciences of the United States of America, 2005, 102 (31): 10898-10903.

[56] HARRIS K S, ZHANG Z, MCMANUS M T, et al. *Dicer* function is essential for lung epithelium morphogenesis [J]. Proceedings of the National Academy of Sciences of the United States of America, 2006, 103 (7): 2208-2213.

[57] YANG W J, YANG D D, NA S, et al. Dicer is required for embryonic angiogenesis during mouse development [J]. The journal of biological chemistry, 2005, 280 (10): 9330-9335.

[58] MULJO S A, ANSEL K M, KANELLOPOULOU C, et al. Aberrant T cell differentiation in the absence of Dicer [J]. The journal of experimental medicine, 2005, 202 (2):

261-269.

[59] AMBROS V. The functions of animal microRNAs [J]. Nature, 2004, 431 (7006): 350-355.

[60] BAGGA S, BRACHT J, HUNTER S, et al. Regulation by *let-7* and *lin-4* miRNAs results in target mRNA degradation [J]. Cell, 2005, 122 (4): 553-563.

[61] HAYASHI K, CHUVA DE SOUSA LOPES S M, KANEDA M, et al. MicroRNA biogenesis is required for mouse primordial germ cell development and spermatogenesis [J]. PLoS one, 2008, 3 (3): e1738.

[62] BARTEL D P. MicroRNAs: genomics, biogenesis, mechanism, and function [J]. Cell, 2004, 116 (2): 281-297.

[63] BARTEL D P, CHEN C Z. Micromanagers of gene expression: the potentially widespread influence of metazoan microRNAs [J]. Nature reviews genetics, 2004, 5 (5): 396-400.

[64] MIRANDA K C, HUYNH T, TAY Y, et al. A pattern-based method for the identification of microRNA binding sites and their corresponding heteroduplexes [J]. Cell, 2006, 126 (6): 1203-1217.

[65] BEREZIKOV E, GURYEV V, VAN DE BELT J, et al. Phylogenetic shadowing and computational identification of human microRNA genes [J]. Cell, 2005, 120 (1): 21-24.

[66] SELBACH M, SCHWANHÄUSSER B, THIERFELDER N, et al. Widespread changes in protein synthesis induced by microRNAs [J]. Nature, 2008, 455 (7209): 58-63.

[67] BAEK D, VILLÉN J, SHIN C, et al. The impact of microRNAs on protein output [J]. Nature, 2008, 455 (7209): 64-71.

[68] BABIARZ J E, BLELLOCH R. Small RNAs-their biogenesis, regulation and function in embryonic stem cells [J]. StemBook, 2009, 3824: 1-16.

[69] JOHN B, ENRIGHT A J, ARAVIN A, et al. Human MicroRNA targets [J]. Plos biology, 2004, 2 (11): e363.

[70] FILIPOWICZ W, BHATTACHARYYA S N, SONENBERG N. Mechanisms of post-transcriptional regulation by microRNAs: are the answers in sight? [J]. Nature reviews genetics, 2008, 9 (2): 102-114.

[71] BEREZIKOV E, CHUNG W J, WILLIS J, et al. Mammalian mirtron genes [J]. Molecular cell, 2007, 28 (2): 328-336.

[72] LUND E, GÜTTINGER S, CALADO A, et al. Nuclear export of microRNA precursors [J]. Science, 2004, 303 (5654): 95-98.

[73] YI R, QIN Y, MACARA I G, et al. Exportin-5 mediates the nuclear export of pre-microRNAs and short hairpin RNAs [J]. Genes & development, 2003, 17 (24): 3011-3016.

[74] SCHWARZ D S, ZAMORE P D. Why do miRNAs live in the miRNP? [J]. Genes &

development, 2002, 16 (9): 1025 - 1031.

[75] GIRALDEZ A J, CINALLI R M, GLASNER M E, et al. MicroRNAs regulate brain morphogenesis in zebrafish [J]. Science, 2005, 308 (5723): 833 - 838.

[76] ZHAO C, SUN G, LI S, et al. A feedback regulatory loop involving microRNA-9 and nuclear receptor TLX in neural stem cell fate determination [J]. Nature structural & molecular biology, 2009, 16 (4): 365 - 371.

[77] HATFIELD S D, SHCHERBATA H R, FISCHER K A, et al. Stem cell division is regulated by the microRNA pathway [J]. Nature, 2005, 435 (7044): 974 - 978.

[78] ALVAREZ-GARCIA I, MISKA E A. MicroRNA functions in animal development and human disease [J]. Development, 2005, 132 (21): 4653 - 4662.

[79] BARBATO C, GIORGI C, CATALANOTTO C, et al. Thinking about RNA? MicroRNAs in the brain [J]. Mammalian genome: Official journal of the International Mammalian Genome Society, 2008, 19 (7 - 8): 541 - 551.

[80] DAVIS T H, CUELLAR T L, KOCH S M, et al. Conditional loss of Dicer disrupts cellular and tissue morphogenesis in the cortex and hippocampus [J]. The journal of neuroscience: the official journal of the Society for Neuroscience, 2008, 28 (17): 4322 - 4330.

[81] GIRALDEZ A J, MISHIMA Y, RIHEL J, et al. Zebrafish MiR-430 promotes deadenylation and clearance of maternal mRNAs [J]. Science, 2006, 312 (5770): 75 - 79.

[82] MISHIMA Y, GIRALDEZ A J, TAKEDA Y, et al. Differential regulation of germline mRNAs in soma and germ cells by zebrafish miR-430 [J]. Current biology, 2006, 16 (21): 2135 - 2142.

[83] ZHAO Y, SAMAL E, SRIVASTAVA D. Serum response factor regulates a muscle-specific microRNA that targets Hand2 during cardiogenesis [J]. Nature, 2005, 436 (7048): 214 - 220.

[84] HARFE B D. MicroRNAs in vertebrate development [J]. Current opinion in genetics & development, 2005, 15 (4): 410 - 415.

[85] BERNSTEIN E, KIM S Y, CARMELL M A, et al. Dicer is essential for mouse development [J]. Nature genetics, 2003, 35 (3): 215 - 217.

[86] WIENHOLDS E, KLOOSTERMAN W P, MISKA E, et al. MicroRNA expression in zebrafish embryonic development [J]. Science, 2005, 309 (5732): 310 - 311.

[87] MCCALLIE B, SCHOOLCRAFT W B, KATZ-JAFFE M G. Aberration of blastocyst microRNA expression is associated with human infertility [J]. Fertility and sterility, 2009, 93: 2374 - 2382.

[88] MAATOUK D M, LOVELAND K L, MCMANUS M T, et al. *Dicer1* is required for differentiation of the mouse male germline [J]. Biology of reproduction, 2008, 79 (4): 696 - 703.

[89] KNIGHT S W, BASS B L. A role for the RNase Ⅲ enzyme DCR-1 in RNA interference

and germ line development in *Caenorhabditis elegans* [J]. Science, 2001, 293 (5538): 2269-2271.

[90] DIEDERICHS S, HABER D A. Dual role for argonautes in microRNA processing and posttranscriptional regulation of microRNA expression [J]. Cell, 2007, 131 (6): 1097-1108.

[91] O'CARROLL D, MECKLENBRAUKER I, DAS P P, et al. A Slicer-independent role for Argonaute 2 in hematopoiesis and the microRNA pathway [J]. Genes & development, 2007, 21 (16): 1999-2004.

[92] LIU J, CARMELL M A, RIVAS F V, et al. Argonaute2 is the catalytic engine of mammalian RNAi [J]. Science, 2004, 305 (5689): 1437-1441.

[93] KURIMOTO K, YABUTA Y, OHINATA Y, et al. An improved single-cell cDNA amplification method for efficient high-density oligonucleotide microarray analysis [J]. Nucleic acids research, 2006, 34 (5): e42.

[94] CROCE C M, CALIN G A. MiRNAs, cancer, and stem cell division [J]. Cell, 2005, 122 (1): 6-7.

[95] TULAY P, SENGUPTA S B. MicroRNA expression and its association with DNA repair in preimplantation embryos [J]. The journal of reproduction and development, 2016, 62 (3): 225-234.

[96] TULAY P, NAJA R P, CASCALES-ROMAN O, et al. Investigation of microRNA expression and DNA repair gene transcripts in human oocytes and blastocysts [J]. Journal of assisted reproduction and genetics, 2015, 32 (12): 1757-1764.

[97] LIU J, VALENCIA-SANCHEZ M A, HANNON G J, et al. MicroRNA-dependent localization of targeted mRNAs to mammalian P-bodies [J]. Nature cell biology, 2005, 7 (7): 719-723.

[98] AMANAI M, BRAHMAJOSYULA M, PERRY A C. A restricted role for sperm-borne microRNAs in mammalian fertilization [J]. Biology of reproduction, 2006, 75 (6): 877-884.

[99] ZOVOILIS A, SMORAG L, PANTAZI A, et al. Members of the miR-290 cluster modulate in vitro differentiation of mouse embryonic stem cells [J]. Differentiation, 2009, 78 (2-3): 69-78.

[100] CHOI W Y, GIRALDEZ A J, SCHIER A F. Target protectors reveal dampening and balancing of Nodal agonist and antagonist by miR-430 [J]. Science, 2007, 318 (5848): 271-274.

[101] YANG Y, BAI W, ZHANG L, et al. Determination of microRNAs in mouse preimplantation embryos by microarray [J]. Developmental dynamics: an official publication of the American Association of Anatomists, 2008, 237 (9): 2315-2327.

[102] NAVARRO A, MONZO M. MicroRNAs in human embryonic and cancer stem cells [J]. Yonsei medical journal, 2010, 51 (5): 622-632.

[103] CHANG T C, WENTZEL E A, KENT O A, et al. Transactivation of miR-34a by p53 broadly influences gene expression and promotes apoptosis [J]. Molecular cell, 2007, 26 (5): 745-752.

[104] RAVER-SHAPIRA N, MARCIANO E, MEIRI E, et al. Transcriptional activation of miR-34a contributes to p53-mediated apoptosis [J]. Molecular cell, 2007, 26 (5): 731-743.

[105] PARÍS R, HENRY R E, STEPHENS S J, et al. Multiple p53-independent gene silencing mechanisms define the cellular response to p53 activation [J]. Cell cycle, 2008, 7 (15): 2427-2433.

[106] LODYGIN D, TARASOV V, EPANCHINTSEV A, et al. Inactivation of miR-34a by aberrant CpG methylation in multiple types of cancer [J]. Cell cycle, 2008, 7 (16): 2591-2600.

[107] MULLER D W, BOSSERHOFF A K. Integrin beta 3 expression is regulated by let-7a miRNA in malignant melanoma [J]. Oncogene, 2008, 27 (52): 6698-6706.

[108] MARTON S, GARCIA M R, ROBELLO C, et al. Small RNAs analysis in CLL reveals a deregulation of miRNA expression and novel miRNA candidates of putative relevance in CLL pathogenesis [J]. Leukemia, 2008, 22 (2): 330-338.

[109] HAYASHITA Y, OSADA H, TATEMATSU Y, et al. A polycistronic microRNA cluster, miR-17-92, is overexpressed in human lung cancers and enhances cell proliferation [J]. Cancer research, 2005, 65 (21): 9628-9632.

[110] DURRUTHY-DURRUTHY J, SEBASTIANO V, WOSSIDLO M, et al. The primate-specific noncoding RNA HPAT5 regulates pluripotency during human preimplantation development and nuclear reprogramming [J]. Nature genetics, 2016, 48 (1): 44-52.

[111] WANG Y, XUE S, LIU X, et al. Analyses of long non-coding RNA and mRNA profiling using RNA sequencing during the pre-implantation phases in pig endometrium [J]. Scientific reports, 2016, 6: 20238.

[112] ANTHONY S, BUITENDIJK S E, DORREPAAL C A, et al. Congenital malformations in 4224 children conceived after IVF [J]. Human reproduction, 2002, 17 (8): 2089-2095.

[113] DEBAUN M R, NIEMITZ E L, FEINBERG A P. Association of in vitro fertilization with Beckwith-Wiedemann syndrome and epigenetic alterations of *LIT1* and *H19* [J]. American journal of human genetics, 2003, 72 (1): 156-160.

[114] WHITE C R, DENOMME M M, TEKPETEY F R, et al. High frequency of imprinted methylation errors in human preim-plantation embryos [J]. Scientific reports, 2015, 5: 17311.

[115] RINAUDO P F, GIRITHARAN G, TALBI S, et al. Effects of oxygen tension on gene expression in preimplantation mouse embryos [J]. Fertility and sterility, 2006, 86

(Suppl 4): 1252 – 1265.

[116] RINAUDO P, SCHULTZ R M. Effects of embryo culture on global pattern of gene expression in preimplantation mouse embryos [J]. Reproduction, 2004, 128 (3): 1 – 11.

[117] GIRITHARAN G, TALBI S, DONJACOUR A, et al. Effect of in vitro fertilization on gene expression and development of mouse preimplantation embryos [J]. Reproduction, 2007, 134 (1): 63 – 72.

[118] GIRITHARAN G, LI M W, DI SEBASTIANO F, et al. Effect of ICSI on gene expression and development of mouse preimplantation embryos [J]. Human reproduction, 2010, 25 (12): 3012 – 3024.

[119] MARKOULAKI S, KUROKAWA M, YOON S Y, et al. Comparison of Ca^{2+} and CaMKII responses in IVF and ICSI in the mouse [J]. Molecular human reproduction, 2007, 13 (4): 265 – 272.

[120] KUROKAWA M, FISSORE R A. ICSI-generated mouse zygotes exhibit altered calcium oscillations, inositol 1, 4, 5-trisphosphate receptor-1 down-regulation, and embryo development [J]. Molecular human reproduction, 2003, 9 (9): 523 – 533.

[121] FERNÁNDEZ-GONZALEZ R, MOREIRA P N, PÉREZ-CRESPO M, et al. Long-term effects of mouse intracytoplasmic sperm injection with DNA-fragmented sperm on health and behavior of adult offspring [J]. Biology of reproduction, 2008, 78 (4): 761 – 772.

(Pinar Tulay)

第6章 通过分析培养基对胚胎存活率进行无创评估

近年来,不孕症在发达国家正发展为一个日益严重的公共卫生问题。辅助生殖技术,特别是体外受精技术,可在一定程度上解决自然生殖率低的问题。如今,单胚胎移植在临床实践中取得了进展,促使人们开发出更可靠的方法来选择最佳胚胎。在传统的临床实践中,移植胚胎的选择是根据形态学评估的。通过检测胚胎在体外培养中用过的培养基中的生物标志物,为进一步的胚胎无创评估提供了非常重要的判断依据。目前的测量方法主要集中在发育中的胚胎的非化合物代谢组学活性上。这些研究主要利用现代分析和蛋白质组学的工具。Montskó 等在 2015 年发表的一篇论文显示,人类结合珠蛋白分子的 α-1 链被认为是胚胎活力的定量生物标志物,在一系列的回顾性实验中,盲法实验取得了 50% 以上的成功率。本章总结了目前可用的代谢组学和蛋白质组学方法作为胚胎活力的无创分子评估指标。

如今,不孕症是影响发达国家夫妇的一个主要公共健康问题(发展中国家的适龄夫妇同样也面临类似的严峻的不孕不育高发病率——编者注)。人类辅助生殖技术(ART),尤其是体外受精(IVF)技术的广泛应用,可帮助越来越多的育龄夫妇实现生育的愿望。目前,3%~4% 的分娩婴儿是经过 IVF 技术实现妊娠出生的,而且这个比例还在继续增加。ART 的可用性是一个非常重要的话题。文化、法律条件、保险/公共资金体系和数据结构不仅会影响每位居民的治疗周期数量,还会影响 ART 的成功率。美国辅助生殖技术国家总结报告显示,2007 年美国共有 142 000 个体外受精周期[1],而 2014 年的最新结果为 208 604 个周期[2]。所采用的 ART 周期类型(分为非捐赠者或卵子捐赠者周期)因女性年龄而异。在大多数情况下,35 岁以下的女性通常使用自己的卵子(非捐赠者卵子),只有约 4% 的女性使用捐赠者卵子。然而,38% 的 43~44 岁女性和 73% 的 44 岁以上女性需要使用捐赠者卵子[2]。与美国类似,欧洲的 ART 周期数量也呈现出增长趋势。2007 年报告的治疗周期数为 493 134 例[3],而 2012 年的报告记录了 640 144 个周期[4]。在 2012 年报告的 452 578 个新鲜周期中,IVF 和卵胞质内单精子注射(ICSI)的比例分别为 139 978(31%)和 312 600(69%)[4]。尽管相关的显微外科技术得到了不断发展(如 ICSI 和一些新的胚胎培养材料的改进),但成功分娩的比例远远低于预期。在 2016 年发布的欧洲体外受精监测报告[4]中,试管婴儿技术的成功分娩的比例为 27.8%～33.8%。

胚胎移植是一个复杂的过程，需要同时具备一个可存活的胚胎和可接受植入的子宫内膜状态，并有效地促进母体和胚胎的相互作用。对于试管授精后的低分娩率来说，只考量女方原因是不正确的。在欧洲，单胚胎移植（SET）的总比例为30%，55%的周期中发生了双胚胎移植，13%的周期中报告了3胚胎移植，1%的周期中移植了4个或更多胚胎。2012年，SET比例最高的国家为瑞典（76.3%），其后依次为芬兰（75.0%）、挪威（60.8%）、比利时（51.1%）、冰岛（49.4%）、捷克共和国（47.4%）、奥地利（46.5%）和丹麦（46.4%）[4]。如今，SET策略在临床实践中取得了进展和认可。选择SET策略的人数正在增加，这促使人们开发出一种可靠的方法来选择最有活力的胚胎，即选择具有最佳着床潜能的胚胎。在传统的ART临床实践中是根据无创形态学评估选择胚胎移植。一些新的形态学参数，如卵裂率、卵裂球形状和对称性，以及适当的滋养外胚层（TE）或内细胞团（ICM）的比例被认为是胚胎有效植入的重要指标。

1 胚胎形态学

最简洁的评价IVF胚胎生存活力的方法是使用显微镜进行目视检查。使用任何侵入性技术进行胚胎细胞活检（如基因筛查）可能会引发一系列伦理问题。胚胎发育最初几天内受到的任何影响都可能对胚胎后期发育产生不良后果。胚胎形态参数的选择部分取决于受精后观察胚胎的时间。

在胚胎发育的第1天，2个原核（间期合子核）的形态可以在一细胞期合子中分级。合子有2个原核，即1个来自卵母细胞的雌性原核和1个来自精子的雄性原核。在第1个胚胎细胞周期的间期结束之前，2个原核保持分离。据报道，在体外胚胎发育的第1天进行核仁筛查可预测妊娠率，但对于这种形态学标记的有效性仍存在一些分歧[5]。

原核破裂的时间点或受精后第1次卵裂的时间（为同一事件）被认为是反映胚胎生殖潜能的指标之一。Fancsovits等[6]报道了原核破裂时间点与临床妊娠和种植率的关系。最早的原核破裂发生在受精后18 h，最晚的原核破裂发生在受精后31 h。相对于原核破裂较晚的胚胎，原核破裂较早的胚胎出现显著较高的临床妊娠率（48.3% vs 27.3%）和种植率（26.5% vs 15.1%）。

在胚胎发育第2天和随后的胚胎体外培育过程中，可评估卵裂球大小、卵裂率和发育中胚胎的形态。质量最好的胚胎在第2天发育到4～5个卵裂球阶段，第3天有7个或更多的卵裂球[5]。卵裂球的数量、胚胎分裂的对称性也被认为是胚胎质量的评价指标。对称卵裂球形状的胚胎比不对称卵裂球形状的胚胎具有更高的种植率。因此，广泛接受的胚胎分裂模式也可以作为预测植入结果的一个指标[7]。

另一个重要的形态可参数是早期胚胎发育时的细胞碎片比例。无论是体外受精还是

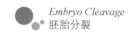

体内受精，任何人类胚胎均可存在细胞碎片比例。胚胎的细胞碎片比例变化很大，从小比例到非常大比例的碎片，甚至出现早期胚胎分裂阶段胚胎严重碎片化，导致卵裂球数量损失。碎片化程度被广泛用作胚胎质量的评估指标和着床潜能的预测指标。广泛碎片化通常与囊胚形成和着床潜能降低有关。如果碎片率低于15%，对囊胚形成似乎没有影响，但超过15%的碎片率会迅速降低囊胚的形成机会[8]。

第5天和第6天胚胎的形态学评分也可通过分析大约十六细胞期分离的内细胞（内细胞团前体）和外细胞（滋养层前体）群体来实现[9]。一个质量较好的囊胚有1个囊胚腔、1个TE和1个ICM组成。因此，检查细胞数量或这些细胞分布区域可能是评估胚胎发育活力的一个重要因素[5]。

从这些例子中也可看出，研究IVF胚胎的形态，利用这些观察结果预测胚胎着床潜能有多种选择。不建议选择单个参数进行评估，而应选择多个参数的组合。为了最大限度地提高评估准确性，需要结合分析合子分级、胚胎分裂阶段和囊胚（如果可能）的完整胚胎发育史来分析[5]。形态学评估是一种成本低廉的评估方法，可以很容易地在临床环境中实现。形态学评估的最大缺点为它是一种高度主观的方法。因此，有必要就这些参数形成共识，即需要使用哪些形态学标记，这些参数在最终分数中的权重是多少，以及所有单个参数的评分标准。2011年，生殖医学领域的科学家和欧洲人类生殖与胚胎学学会（European Society for Human Reproduction and Embryology，ESHRE）胚胎学特别兴趣小组根据不同发育阶段的若干形态学标记达成了一项国际共识。该共识的结果称为伊斯坦布尔共识计分系统。与胚胎形态评估相关的实验室实践的标准化将有利于提高IVF的治疗效果。Alpha科学家小组制定的文件旨在为准确描述胚胎发育提供全球标准化共识[10]。伊斯坦布尔共识计分系数由多个形态学评估参数组成，同时还需考虑受精后的对应事件发生时间。如今，这些指南集已成为IVF胚胎生存能力评估的公认方法。

2　胚胎培养基的分析

由于伦理原因，人们一直在努力寻找无创方法来评估胚胎的生存能力。通过分析胚胎分泌的化合物或通过研究胚胎在培养基中的变化来研究胚胎的代谢活性是一种直接的办法。培养基对于胚胎环境有重要影响，可维持单胚胎移植目标的实现，是维持可接受的妊娠率的关键，因此选择最佳培养基是一个关键点。

第一批人类胚胎在简单盐溶液中培养，或在最初设计用于组织培养的较复杂的培养基中培养。这些早期培养基是由葡萄糖、丙酮酸和乳酸的生理盐溶液组成，并补充患者血清。后来研究发现，在培养基中添加氨基酸可提高生殖潜能。动物和人类模型的研究结果都显示氨基酸的引入对胚胎发育有积极影响，并提高了胚胎体外生存能力[11]。

借助文献中分享的经验，一些诊所开始开发"内部"胚胎培养基；但通过这种方式开发的培养基和培养环境的标准化并非易事[11]。因此，为满足日益增长的需求而专门设计用于临床 IVF 应用的商业化培养基很快就被开发出来。这些培养基是在标准化条件、法规和质量控制下在专业工厂中无菌生产的，因此是"内部"胚胎培养基的一个有吸引力的替代品。目前，存在两种类型的商业培养基：序贯培养基和"一步法"培养基。"一步法"培养基使用单一培养基成分来支持合子发育到囊胚阶段。"一步法"培养基的局限性在于它不能适应胚胎发育过程中不断变化的生化需求：适合早期卵裂状态胚胎的培养基成分可能不适合囊胚期胚胎，因此，大多数 IVF 诊所使用序贯培养基。已有文献确定，支持囊胚发育的条件可能会抑制早期卵裂期胚胎的发育。如果临床实践中包括囊胚培养和囊胚移植，序贯培养基是最佳选择[11]。

人血清白蛋白是任何类型胚胎培养基的重要的添加剂，它是血液中最丰富的可溶性蛋白质成分，具有多种生理作用。在培养基中，白蛋白充当 pH 缓冲液、渗透调节剂、膜稳定剂、表面活性剂和金属或有毒物质的清除剂。早些时候，白蛋白是从人或母体血清中获取的，但现在已转向使用纯化白蛋白产品，其主要原因是前者具有传播传染病的风险，使用纯化白蛋白产品可以消除这种风险。然而，不同批次的白蛋白产品的稳定性难以保证。重组白蛋白的使用可解决上述所有问题，但其使用不如纯化白蛋白产品广泛[12]。

当使用纯化的白蛋白产品时，必须考虑到这些产品的纯度并不是 100% 的。Dyrlund 等[13]最近的研究显示，在含有纯化人血清白蛋白产品的市售培养基中鉴定出除白蛋白以外的 110 种蛋白质。这些培养基已经使用了几十年，对临床并无明确害处，也许在临床实践中不是一个严重的问题，然而，如果我们将该培养基用作研究材料，这是一个非常重要的需要考量的问题。

培养后培养液的测量可作为寻找胚胎活力标志物的一种特殊的无创替代方法。在培养基中，化合物可分为两大类：一类由存在于一般培养基中的化合物组成，这些化合物可被发育中的胚胎定量改变（如营养素或肽/蛋白质化合物）[14]；另一类是胚胎分泌到周围培养基中的胚胎相关分子（如蛋白质和代谢终产物）。为了分析发育中胚胎的分泌体（尤其是蛋白质），必须了解哪些已识别的蛋白质来源于胚胎，哪些蛋白质本来存在于普通培养基，或者只是蛋白质的浓度在何时发生何种变化。

3 代谢组学研究

目前，IVF 的目标是减少移植周期内胚胎的数目，最好实现单胚胎移植。因此，越来越需要新的胚胎生存能力标志物以确定待移植胚胎。葡萄糖摄取率或培养基中丙酮酸浓度已被确定为植入胚胎发育潜能的合适的生物标志物。小鼠模型和人类研究的结果显示，植入子宫后正常发育的囊胚在体外培养时的葡萄糖消耗率显著高于未植入的囊胚[15-16]。在人类胚胎的体外发育过程中，形成正常囊胚的胚胎对丙酮酸和葡萄糖的摄取量明显高于不能正常发育的胚胎。正常发育组每个胚胎每小时葡萄糖摄取量平均为

22.1 pmol，非正常发育组每个胚胎每小时葡萄糖摄取量仅为 10.2 pmol。比较不同形态分级的胚胎的葡萄糖摄取量发现，最高等级的囊胚葡萄糖摄取量最高。在同一患者的同一级别囊胚中，葡萄糖摄取量显著增加，这表明体外发育过程中的葡萄糖消耗量是胚胎活力的关键信息。相关研究还表明，培养基中葡萄糖的测量比丙酮酸的测量更重要，丙酮酸的摄取量与囊胚发育级别无关。

氨基酸在胚胎发育早期具有多种生物学功能。可以对培养基中的氨基酸成分进行定量分析，以检查早期胚胎发育期间的氨基酸变迁。Houghton 等[17]使用高效液相色谱法对单个人类胚胎的氨基酸变迁进行了定量分析，发现能继续形成囊胚的胚胎和未能发育到囊胚阶段的胚胎有不同的氨基酸利用模式。在正常发育的胚胎组中，培养基中亮氨酸的消耗量增加。研究还发现，丙氨酸、精氨酸、谷氨酰胺、蛋氨酸和天冬酰胺的分布可以显著预测胚胎的发育潜能。Brison 等[18]揭示了培养到二细胞期的人类合子培养基中氨基酸浓度的变化，发现天冬酰胺、甘氨酸和亮氨酸 3 种氨基酸的转换与临床妊娠和活产显著相关。

胚胎发育潜能指标不仅可以通过分析选定的代谢组化合物，还可以通过分析总代谢组变化来揭示。代谢组学实验可检查培养基的整体代谢物含量，而不仅仅测量已知的营养素或代谢物。使用拉曼光谱或近红外光谱等分析技术，可以获得胚胎培养基的整个光谱轮廓。必须强调的是，该方法不能识别特定成分，只能检测所获得光谱的特定变化。这种方法的潜在优势是可以对培养基环境进行全面分析[19]。该方法得以实现的原理是：在具有不同植入结果的胚胎培养基样品中进行多波长光谱分析，寻找光谱变化；利用数学算法将这些差异计算得到胚胎生存能力得分或指数。观察到的光谱变化是由于胚胎代谢活动导致的化学基团数量的差异。该方法无法确定造成光谱差异的特定化合物，但可以间接报告发育中胚胎代谢组学活性的信息。例如，如果近红外光谱特征在 750～950 nm 光谱区域显示出差异，则报告—OH、—CH 和—NH 基团相对数量的变化[20]。对已知具有着床潜能的胚胎的残余培养基进行的拉曼光谱和近红外光谱分析表明，代表临床妊娠的移植胚胎的存活指数较高。当使用红外光谱法检查具有相似形态的胚胎时，存活率得分显著不同，这表明对总代谢组的分析也显示了胚胎存活率的额外信息[19]。研究结果表现，体外受精胚胎培养基的无创代谢组学分析在胚胎发育潜能评估过程中占有一席之地。也许一种新的方法无法取代现有的形态学评估方法，然而它可以通过识别形态学评估未注意到的生物标志物来增加部分低种植率胚胎的相关信息。

4　蛋白质组学研究

据推测，在培养基中发现的分泌性化合物可提供胚胎特征性的分子指纹，这些信息可以告诉我们与胚胎生长、发育能力和着床潜能相关的信息。随着敏感和特殊的新分析技术的出现，对植入前胚胎周围环境进行全面分析成为可能[21]。这些分子图谱应该能够高精度地区分活胚胎和非活胚胎的差异[22]。鉴定胚胎分泌的新生物标志物可以显著提高体外受精周期的效率，提高每次移植的妊娠率，降低手术成本。更可靠的胚胎生存能力评估还有一个更重要的作用，即减少患者的情绪压力[23]。生物功能通常由蛋白质调节或执行，因此了解单个细胞或一小群细胞的功能是至关重要的。蛋白质组的分析显示了胚胎对外部和内部条件的反应。对胚胎培养基的蛋白质进行分析，为早期胚胎发育过程中激活的生化途径提供了新的分子鉴定视角[21]。

  胚胎分泌的蛋白质组学分析使用的最新分析工具一般包括质谱（mass spectrometry，MS）或液相色谱-质谱（liquid chromatography-mass spectrometry，LC-MS）。其中，MS可能是研究胚胎分泌体最有希望的技术。标准蛋白质组学分析方法包括使用2D凝胶电泳分离完整蛋白质，然后立即进行MS分析；或者通过消化，随后分析产生的肽谱。对试验和对照的胚胎培养基采用胰蛋白酶消化随后行LC-MS分析，胚胎相关肽和蛋白质的变化也成为一种分析方法。纳米级超高效液相色谱（nano-ultra-high erformance liquid chromatography，nano-UPLC）和MS的无标签定量方法，允许在一次分析过程中使用最少数量的样品，并有效识别大量肽和蛋白质[24]。基质辅助激光解吸电离飞行时间质谱（matrix-assisted laser desorption ionization time of flight，MALDI-TOF）和表面增强激光解吸电离飞行时间质谱（surface-enhanced laser desorption ionization time of flight，SELDI-TOF）也可用于检测胚胎培养基中的不同蛋白质成分或浓度。SELDI-TOF是一种重要且高度敏感的高通量蛋白质组学分析方法，尤其对于低分子量蛋白质分析更为有效[21]。

  胚胎分泌的活性候选标志物涵盖了多种分子。Sher等[25]使用可溶性人类白细胞抗原G（sHLA-G）作为胚胎种植率和妊娠率的预测因子。使用免疫分析法对sHLA-G进行定量分析，并根据定量结果将胚胎分为2组，高于几何平均数的sHLA-G的胚胎被视为sHLA-G$^+$，而低于几何平均数的sHLA-G的胚胎被视为sHLA-G$^-$。在sHLA-G$^+$组中，观察到明显较高的种植率和妊娠率。sHLA-G$^+$组的种植率和妊娠率分别为44%和75%，而sHLA-G$^-$组的种植率和妊娠率分别为14%和23%。

  相关文献[26]也描述了载脂蛋白A1在胚胎发育中的关联作用，通过凝胶电泳和MALDI-TOF进行鉴定，以及酶联免疫吸附测定（enzyme-linked immunosorbent assay，ELISA）和定量逆转录聚合酶链反应（quantitatiue reverse transcriptase poly-metase chain reaction，qRT-PCR）对载脂蛋白A1的mRNA进行定量。研究发现载脂蛋白A1水平与囊胚分级相关，但与种植率和妊娠率无关。与这些发现相反，Nyalwidhe等[22]使用MS、蛋白质印迹法（western blotting，western-blot）和ELISA鉴定了14种不同的调节肽，这些肽随后被用于通过遗传关联算法来区分胚胎移植成功周期与失败周期。这种遗传关联算法能够以71%～84%的准确率识别胚胎移植周期中的妊娠率。在这14种肽中，有几个被鉴定为载脂蛋白A1的片段，在培养基样本中表达量减少，从而导致胚胎种植率降低。McReynolds等[27]报道了一种基于蛋白质组学分析的有趣方法：使用串联质谱（MS/MS）模式下运行的线性四极傅里叶变换（linear trap quadropole-fourier transform，LTQ-FT）超混合质谱仪选择潜在的生物标志物候选物。利用这一蛋白质组学平台，鉴定出了lipocalin-1与染色体非整倍体的相关性。使用市售lipocalin-1 ELISA试剂盒测定lipocalin-1的浓度。根据微滴培养基中lipocalin-1浓度的变化，可以明确区分整倍体和非整倍体胚胎。非整倍体囊胚的 lipocalin-1 浓度比整倍体囊胚的浓度增加更为显著。汇集的微滴整倍体胚胎含有 3～4 ng/mL 的 lipocalin-1，而非整倍体胚胎含有浓度为 6～7 ng/mL 的该化合物。分析残余培养基样品，单个微滴的整倍体和非整倍体胚胎时，结果分别为 4～5 ng/mL 和 5～6 ng/mL 的 lipocalin-1。

这些研究清楚地表明，对残余培养基样品进行无创蛋白质组学分析，对于确定胚胎发育潜能具有巨大潜能。因此，该方法可以整合到现有胚胎评估体系中。

5 使用结合珠蛋白 α-1 链的定量测定评估胚胎生存能力

通过对培养 3 天的残余培养基样品进行 LC-MS 分析，检测到 4 种不同的多肽，质谱显示 4 种多肽的单同位素质量分别为 4 787.4 Da、4 464.6 Da、4 622.4 Da 和 9 186.5 Da，显示了存活（成功妊娠）和非存活（未妊娠）胚胎组之间的差异[28]，经过多种蛋白质组学和统计学分析，最终候选了生物标志物为 9 186.5 Da 的多肽。相应的质谱图如图 6-1 所示。

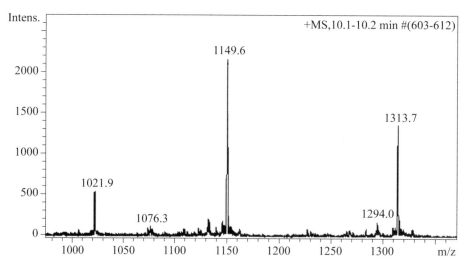

横轴表示质量/电荷（m/z），纵轴表示绝对峰值强度。m/z 1 149.6 处的最强峰对应于分子的 $^{[m+8H]}$8+ 离子峰，m/z 1 021.9 和 m/z 1 313.7 处的峰分别代表分子的 $^{[m+9H]}$9+ 离子峰和 $^{[m+7H]}$7+ 离子峰。

图 6-1　结合珠蛋白 α-1 片段的质谱

在活胚胎组和非活胚胎组中，只有结合珠蛋白 α-1 片段在数量上存在显著性差异（$P = 0.005$）。在消化各色谱组分后进行蛋白质组学鉴定。通过使用 MS 数据，进行数据库搜索和手动检索条目的序列注释，该蛋白质被确定为人类结合珠蛋白的 α-1 链。该亚单位的 α-1 形式具有 9 186.4 Da 的单同位素质量。通过串联质谱鉴定，所有酶片段都对应于结合珠蛋白前体蛋白区域。

在一组盲法和回顾性实验中，包括对 161 个结合珠蛋白 α-1 链进行测量，发现 62 个样本在生物化学上不可检，99 个样本在生物化学上可检。生化不可检的 62 个胚胎均未成功分娩，而生化可检组的妊娠率为 55%（图 6-2）。结果显示，在 α-1 链数量差异的基础上，存活胚胎组和非存活胚胎组之间存在显著性差异（$P<0.001$）。此外，发现肽片段的数量与妊娠结局之间存在显著相关性（$P<0.001$）。

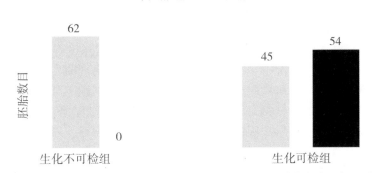

在被评估为生化不可检的组中，未发现妊娠。经生物化学鉴定为生化可检的存活胚胎组，其妊娠率为 55%（图片中为 54%）。

图 6-2　培养 3 天后胚胎培养基的盲法分析结果（$n=161$）

在一般培养基中，人类结合珠蛋白的可能来源是各种纯化蛋白产物的蛋白质污染。培养基中结合珠蛋白 α-1 链是由于连接成熟结合珠蛋白分子链的二硫键减少产生的。非存活胚胎样本中 α-1 链数量增加的原因可能是异常发育或受损的胚胎通常比正常胚胎表现出更大程度的凋亡特征。细胞凋亡随后可能伴随继发性坏死和膜通透性增加。我们假设这些过程可导致酶或其他化学因子从异常发育的胚胎细胞中介入，从而改变胚胎培养基中的化学环境。

6　胚胎早期发育中的细胞凋亡

细胞程序性死亡（programmed cell death，PCD）也称为细胞凋亡，是一种常见的生物学现象。它以细胞膜起泡、染色质浓缩和 DNA 断裂为特征，涉及多种膜受体和信号转导通路的激活。细胞凋亡的典型标志是细胞收缩、核浓缩和称为"凋亡小体"的小泡的形成。与细胞凋亡相关的最重要的生化事件是 DNA 断裂，产生一种称为 DNA 碎片的特异性凝胶电泳图像。细胞凋亡发生在每个多细胞生物体中，是一个重要的生物学过程[29]。

早期胚胎的正常细胞凋亡对胚胎正常发育至关重要。例如，在囊胚中，内细胞团和滋养外胚层都会发生凋亡[29]。植入前胚胎正常发育过程中的细胞凋亡具有多种功能。

据推测，胚泡内部的细胞数量遵循一种平衡，细胞凋亡有助于维持细胞内稳态。早期胚胎发育中细胞凋亡错误的另一个可能原因是，基因结构异常改变的细胞或具有其他异常或发育潜能不足的细胞被清除。例如，在内细胞团中，非整倍体细胞的出现是广泛存在的，非整倍体细胞可通过细胞凋亡完成清除，从而维持正常细胞的发育。凋亡标志物也被认为是卵母细胞和胚胎质量评估的重要附加特征之一。停滞发育的胚胎往往具有高度的凋亡特征[30]。

凋亡细胞通常应被吞噬，如果凋亡细胞不被吞噬，它们可能会发生继发性坏死。坏死与凋亡不同，坏死主要表现为细胞膜通透性增加、胞浆结构排泄增加。这些事件在各种不同的细胞类型中均可观察到[31]。凋亡程序提供了两种细胞消除的替代方法。早期表面信号可使吞噬细胞识别凋亡细胞，并通过"沉默"清除过程将其清除。继发性坏死发生在缺乏吞噬细胞的情况下，导致最终的自溶解体。出现凋亡的细胞表现出特定的凋亡迹象和坏死特征，如细胞质膜的降解。当功能性吞噬细胞不可用时，继发性坏死也可能在体内发生，并伴有一些病理情况出现[32]。体外细胞凋亡倾向于以类似的方式进行，包括水解酶的激活和细胞质膜的损伤，从而导致细胞裂解。如果去除凋亡细胞或凋亡小体过程失败，就会发生上述过程。原发性坏死过程中描述的事件也在继发性坏死过程中起作用。细胞死亡的机制涉及蛋白酶活性引起的蛋白质水解，导致细胞溶质化合物的额外释放[33]。对动物模型的研究表明，体外培养可增加细胞凋亡，并且培养基的组成可影响该过程的发生率，原因是培养基缺乏一些关键的母体"生存"因素[31]。在体外培养过程中观察到细胞凋亡增加，推测是由于人工体外环境中缺乏清除细胞过程，导致发生继发性坏死。结合珠蛋白断裂现象是因继发性坏死和膜通透性增加导致胚胎细胞释放因子所致。

7 结论

我们的详细研究表明，人类结合珠蛋白分子的 α-1 链可用作区分体外培养胚胎植入能力的生物标志物，而其他人此前尚未证明这是胚胎活力的指标。生化不可检的胚胎不会引起妊娠，而生化可检组的胚胎显示有 55% 的妊娠率。研究中，没有测定结合珠蛋白 α-1 片段的对照组仅有 30% 的妊娠率。无创代谢组学和蛋白质组学方法可在常规体外受精过程中占有一席之地，但不能完全替代形态学评估过程。理想的体外受精可包括这一步骤：排除形态最差的胚胎，然后在实验室测量剩余胚胎培养基的结合珠蛋白 α-1 链量的多少。这项技术的主要缺点是：需要在常规体外受精过程中应用质谱技术，但多数生殖中心通常不具备这种昂贵的实验室设备。芯片实验室概念的发展与现有的医疗器械相结合，可能成为一个胚胎活性检测的爆发点[34]。

致谢

本研究得到匈牙利科学研究基金——OTKA/115394/2015/HU "胚胎活力的早期生

化指标", EDIOP-2.3.2-15-2016-00021/HU "芯片技术在提高人类体外受精效率中的应用"的支持, 也得到匈牙利佩奇大学实施智能专业化战略项目 EPop-3.61.-16-2016-00004 和 úNKP-17-4-Ⅲ "人力资源部国新卓越计划"的资助。

参考文献

[1] SELI E, SAKKAS D, SCOTT R, et al. Noninvasive metabolomic profiling of embryo culture media using Raman and near-infrared spectroscopy correlates with reproductive potential of embryos in women undergoing in vitro fertilization [J]. Fertility and sterility, 2007, 88 (5): 1350-1357.

[2] 2014 Assisted Reproductive Technology National Summary Report [EB/OL]. [2016-10]. https://www.cdc.gov/art/pdf/2014-report/art-2014-national-summary-report.pdf.

[3] DE MOUZON J, GOOSSENS V, BHATTACHARYA S, et al. Assisted reproductive technology in Europe, 2007: results generated from European registers by ESHRE [J]. Human reproduction, 2012, 27 (4): 954-966.

[4] European IVF-Monitoring Consortium (EIM) for the European Society of Human Reproduction and Embryology (ESHRE), CALHAZ-JORGE C, DE GEYTER C, et al. Assisted reproductive technology in Europe, 2012: results generated from European registers by ESHRE [J]. Human reproduction, 2016, 31 (8): 1638-1652.

[5] AJDUK A, ZERNICKA-GOETZ M. Quality control of embryo development [J]. Molecular aspects of medicine, 2013, 34 (5): 903-918.

[6] FANCSOVITS P, TOTH L, TAKACS Z F, et al. Early pronuclear breakdown is a good indicator of embryo quality and viability [J]. Fertility and sterility, 2005, 84 (4): 881-887.

[7] SELA R, SAMUELOV L, ALMOG B, et al. An embryo cleavage pattern based on the relative blastomere size as a function of cell number for predicting implantation outcome [J]. Fertility and sterility, 2012, 98 (3): 650-656.

[8] HARDY K, STARK J, WINSTON R M L. Maintenance of the inner cell mass in human blastocysts from fragmented embryos [J]. Biology of reproduction, 2003, 68 (4): 1165-1169.

[9] BOISO I, VEIGA A, EDWARDS R G. Fundamentals of human embryonic growth in vitro and the selection of high-quality embryos for transfer [J]. Reproductive biomedicine online, 2002, 5 (3): 328-350.

[10] ALPHA Scientists in Reproductive Medicine, ESHRE Special Interest Group Embryology. Istanbul consensus workshop on embryo assessment: proceedings of an expert meeting [J]. Reproductive biomedicine online, 2011, 22 (6): 632-646.

[11] LANE M, GARDNER D K. Embryo culture medium: which is the best? [J]. Best practice & research clinical obstetrics & gynaecology, 2007, 21 (1): 83-100.

[12] BLAKE D, SVALANDER P, JIN M, et al. Protein supplementation of human IVF cul-

ture media [J]. Journal of assisted reproduction and genetics, 2002, 19 (3): 137 – 143.

[13] DYRLUND T F, KIRKEGAARD K, POULSEN E T, et al. Unconditioned commercial embryo culture media contain a large variety of non-declared proteins: A comprehensive proteomics analysis [J]. Human reproduction, 2014, 29 (11): 2421 – 2430.

[14] RØDGAARD T, HEEGAARD P M H, CALLESEN H. Non-invasive assessment of invitro embryo quality to improve transfer success [J]. Reproductive biomedicine online, 2015, 31 (5): 585 – 592.

[15] GARDNER D K, WALE P L. Analysis of metabolism to select viable human embryos for transfer [J]. Fertility and sterility, 2013, 99 (4): 1062 – 1072.

[16] GARDNER D K, LANE M, STEVENS J, et al. Non-invasive assessment of human embryo nutrient consumption as a measure of developmental potential [J]. Fertility and sterility, 2001, 76 (6): 1175 – 1180.

[17] HOUGHTON F D, HAWKHEAD J A, HUMPHERSON P G, et al. Non-invasive amino acid turnover predicts human embryo developmental capacity [J]. Human reproduction, 2002, 17 (4): 999 – 1005.

[18] BRISON D R, HOUGHTON F D, FALCONER D, et al. Identification of viable embryos in IVF by non-invasive measurement of amino acid turnover [J]. Human reproduction, 2004, 19 (10): 2319 – 2324.

[19] VERGOUW C G, BOTROS L L, JUDGE K, et al. Non-invasive viability assessment of day-4 frozen-thawed human embryos using near infrared spectroscopy [J]. Reproductive biomedicine online, 2011, 23 (6): 769 – 776.

[20] SELI E, SAKKAS D, SCOTT R, et al. Non-invasive metabolomic profiling of embryo culture media using Raman and near-infrared spectroscopy correlates with reproductive potential of embryos in women undergoing in vitro fertilization [J]. Fertility and sterility, 2007, 88 (5): 1350 – 1357.

[21] KATZ-JAFFE M G, SCHOOLCRAFT W B, GARDNER D K. Analysis of protein expression (secretome) by human and mouse preimplantation embryos [J]. Fertility and sterility, 2006, 86 (3): 678 – 685.

[22] NYALWIDHE J, BURCH T, BOCCA S, et al. The search for biomarkers of human embryo developmental potential in IVF: a comprehensive proteomic approach [J]. Molecular human reproduction, 2013, 19 (4): 250 – 263.

[23] POLI M, ORI A, CHILD T, et al. Characterization and quantification of proteins secreted by single human embryos prior to implantation [J]. EMBO molecular medicine, 2015, 7 (11): 1465 – 1479.

[24] CORTEZZI S S, GARCIA J S, FERREIRA C R, et al. Secretome of the preimplantation human embryo by bottom-up label-free proteomics [J]. Analytical and bioanalytical chemistry, 2011, 401 (4): 1331 – 1339.

[25] SHER G, KESKINTEPE L, FISCH J D, et al. Soluble human leukocyte antigen G expression in phase I culture media at 46 hours after fertilization predicts pregnancy and implantation from day 3 embryo transfer [J]. Fertility and sterility, 2005, 83 (5): 1410 – 1413.

[26] MAINS L M, CHRISTENSON L, YANG B, et al. Identification of apolipoprotein A1 in the human embryonic secretome [J]. Fertility and sterility, 2011, 96 (2): 422 – 427.

[27] MCREYNOLDS S, VANDERLINDEN L, STEVENS J, et al. Lipocalin-1: A potential marker for non-invasive aneuploidy screening [J]. Fertility and sterility, 2011, 95 (8): 2631 – 2633.

[28] MONTSKÓ G, ZRÍNYI Z, JANÁKY T, et al. Non-invasive embryo viability assessment by quantitation of human haptoglobin alpha-1 fragment in the in vitro fertilization culture medium: an additional tool to increase success rate [J]. Fertility and sterility, 2015, 103 (3): 687 – 693.

[29] BRILL A, TORCHINSKY A, CARP H, et al. The role of apoptosis in normal and abnormal embryonic development [J]. Journal of assisted reproduction and genetics, 1999, 16 (10): 512 – 519.

[30] HAOUZI D, HAMAMAH S. Pertinence of apoptosis markers for the improvement of *in vitro* fertilization (IVF) [J]. Current medical chemistry, 2009, 16 (15): 1905 – 1916.

[31] HARDY K. Apoptosis in the human embryo [J]. Reviews of reproduction, 1999, 4 (3): 125 – 134.

[32] SILVA M T. Secondary necrosis: the natural outcome of the complete apoptotic program [J]. FEBS letters, 2010, 584 (22): 4491 – 4499.

[33] SILVA M T, DO VALE A, DOS SANTOS N M N. Secondary necrosis in multicellular animals: an outcome of apoptosis with pathogenic implications [J]. Apoptosis. 2008, 13 (4): 463 – 482.

[34] LE GAC S, NORDHOFF V. Microfluidics for mammalian embryo culture and selection: Where do we stand now? [J]. Molecular human reproduction, 2017, 23 (4): 213 – 226.

(Gergely Montskó, Zita Zrínyi, ákos Várnagy, József Bódis and Gábor L. Kovács)

第 7 章　两种不同类型培养基和两种不同款型培养箱协同作用改善辅助生殖技术妊娠结局

> 培养基和培养箱对胚胎质量起着关键作用。我们发现不同患者的胚胎对培养基和/或培养箱有不同的响应。将患者的 1 850 个合子随机分为 2 组，分别在 Global 培养基和 P1 培养基中培养，记录卵裂率和胚胎质量。结果表明，第 2 天和第 3 天的卵裂、优质胚胎在不同培养基之间没有统计学差异，但是 45% 的患者胚胎在 2 种培养基中均生长良好；22% 的患者胚胎在 Global 培养基中生长良好，但在 P1 培养基中质量较差；而 21% 的患者胚胎在 P1 培养基中生长良好，但在 Global 培养基中质量较差；只有 12% 的患者胚胎在这两种培养基中生长均不好。P1 培养基组的妊娠率仅为 40%，Global 培养基组的妊娠率为 42.5%（$P > 0.05$），但当两种培养基同时使用时，妊娠率可提高到 70.1%。此外，使用两种培养箱的妊娠率显著高于使用一种培养箱（73.2% vs 60%，$P < 0.05$）。总之，不同患者的胚胎对培养基和培养箱的响应结果表明，使用两种培养基和两种培养箱进行胚胎培养可以显著提高胚胎质量和妊娠率。

辅助生殖技术（ART）（主要包括 IVF 和 ICSI）现已广泛用于不孕不育症的治疗。人类 IVF 的成功应用主要得益于胚胎培养环境（包括培养基和培养箱）的创新改善。迄今为止，不同的培养系统已被成功地用于人和动物胚胎的体外生产。

1912 年首次实现兔胚胎体外培养[1-2]；1956 年，实现了小鼠受精卵在复合培养基中培养至囊胚期[3]。1985 年，一种被称为人类输卵管液（human tubal fluid medium，HTF）培养基的胚胎培养基首次成为人类 IVF 特有培养基[4]。自 HTF 培养基开发以来，人类胚胎培养基的配方进行了许多改进和完善。

几十年来，优化培养基以支持人类和动物胚胎发育一直是科学家关注的焦点[5]。随着对输卵管和子宫生理变化以及卵裂期和囊胚期胚胎不同代谢需求的进一步认知，许多新型胚胎培养基被不断开发。目前，市场上有 3 种类型培养基：①具有附加能量基质的简单盐溶液，如 KSOM、P1 等[6-7]；②复合组织培养基，如 Ham 的 F-10[8]；③序贯培养基，如 G1/G2，以及升级的 G5 培养基[9]。最近的序贯培养基还考虑了胚胎从卵裂到囊胚阶段不断变化的代谢需求[10-11]。目前，许多商业胚胎培养基可用于人类胚胎培养，其对胚胎培养的影响是多种多样的[12]。在 google.com 上搜索关键词"人类胚胎培养基比较"会出现 53 600 个结果。比较这些培养基对胚胎发育影响的研究报告,发现其中有大量相互矛盾的结论。许多研究没有发现不同培养基之间存在显著差异或只有微小差异[13-14]。最近,Mantikou 等[15]使用荟萃分析对 20 种不同培养基的 31 种不同比较方法进行了评估,没有发现不同培养基导致 IVF/ICSI 的妊娠结局存在显著差异。

由于人类胚胎培养基商业公司都在不断提高其现有培养基的质量,因此各种胚胎培养基之间的显著差异可能很难证明。目前,大多数的商业培养基均可以产生令人满意的人类胚胎培养结果。因此,最佳胚胎培养基的选择取决于胚胎学家的兴趣及其特定的工作条件。

此外,IVF 实验室的培养箱在提供优化胚胎发育和临床结局所需的稳定和适当的培养环境方面发挥着关键作用。随着技术的进步,几种类型的培养箱已被应用于 IVF 实验室。最近,Swain[16]对人类体外受精实验室中的胚胎培养箱进行了比较分析,并回顾了一些培养箱的功能、关键环境变量的控制和各个培养单元中使用的技术。这一比较研究表明,较小的台式/顶置培养箱能够更快地恢复环境变量;但对临床结局的分析表明,没有任何特定培养箱具有明显的优势。

根据我们 IVF 中心过去 10 多年的实践,认为 Cook 台式培养箱(顶置开关的小型台式培养箱)和 Forma 水套 CO_2 培养箱(前门开关的大体积培养箱)在胚胎培养方面没有任何差异。但我们也观察到,同一患者的同胞胚胎分别放在两种培养基和两种培养箱条件下,通常具有不同的发育结果。那么,患者的胚胎是否会有对培养基或培养箱条件选择的倾向性?本研究的目的即是确定在人类胚胎培养系统中,患者胚胎对培养基和培养箱的反应是否存在特异性差异。

1 材料和方法

1.1 培养基

本研究主要使用两种培养基进行胚胎培养:P1 培养基(加利福尼亚州欧文科学公司),Global 培养基(加拿大 Life Global 有限责任公司)。两种培养基中均添加 10% 血清替代补充剂(Irvine Scientific, Inc, CA)用于胚胎培养。

1.2 培养箱

本研究主要使用两种培养箱进行胚胎培养:Forma 水套 CO_2 培养箱(Thermal Forma Scientific 公司),连接至医用级 CO_2 气罐,并调整 CO_2 浓度为 5% 用于胚胎培养;Cook 台式培养箱,连接至经认证的预混合三气体罐,其中含有 5% 的 O_2、6% 的 CO_2 和 89% 的 N_2(图 7-1)。尽管两个培养箱连接的 CO_2 浓度不同,但其 pH 测试结果均为 7.21~

7.38；并且在两种类型的培养箱中，两种培养基之间未观察到显著性差异。

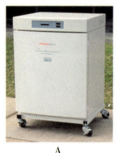
A.

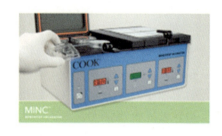
B.

A. 5% CO_2 Forma 水套 CO_2 培养箱；B. 三通气（6% CO_2、5% O_2、89% N_2）Cook 台式培养箱

图 7-1　胚胎培养箱

2　实验设计

这是一项前瞻性随机研究，研究对象是 2012—2013 年在美国亚利桑那州生殖医学研究中心接受辅助生殖技术治疗的不孕夫妇。在此期间，所有患者（年龄 25～43 岁）在提取卵母细胞之前均接受了我们的标准刺激方案（LA/HMG，HCG 10 000 IU/mL）治疗。取卵术后将卵母细胞置于 P1 培养基（Irvine Scientific，Inc）和 3% 人血清白蛋白（HSA，In-VitoCare，Frederick，MD）中，在 37℃ 5% CO_2 培养箱中培养 4～6 h。然后，根据精子质量（约 35% 的周期需要 ICSI），将卵母细胞常规放置于 100 μL P1 培养基微滴中进行 IVF，或通过 ICSI 受精。第二天，即 IVF 或 ICSI 后 18～20 h 评估受精情况。如果观察到 2 个不同的原核（2PN），则确认受精。将每位患者的受精卵随机分为 2 组，并在培养皿中的 P1 培养基或 Life Global 培养基中培养，每滴 50 μL 培养基再培养 2 天（图 7-2）。

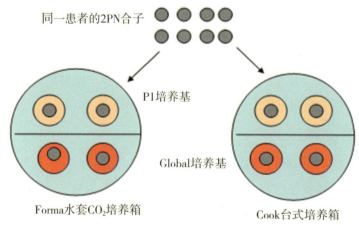

图 7-2　胚胎培养方法

第7章 两种不同类型培养基和两种不同款型培养箱协同作用改善辅助生殖技术妊娠结局

一名患者的同胞受精合子被随机置于两种培养基和两种培养箱中进行培养。

每个胚胎均在一个单独的微滴中培养。体外培养 24 h 和 48 h 后，评估胚胎卵裂状态和胚胎发育质量。由至少 2 位经验丰富的胚胎学家在倒置显微镜上放大 100 倍进行观察，根据卵裂球的数量、大小均等性、是否存在颗粒感以及核碎片的相对比例来评估胚胎等级。根据我们的标准，优质或顶级胚胎（5 级）被定义为细胞外碎片少于 10% 的规则球形卵裂球，第 3 天有 6～10 个卵裂球。1～4 级胚胎被定义为低质量胚胎。胚胎移植当天，根据患者年龄和胚胎质量，选择 1～4 个胚胎进行腹部超声引导下移植到子宫。记录每种培养基或培养箱中的移植胚胎。从两种培养基和两种培养箱中选择质量好的胚胎进行移植，将剩下的胚胎留在培养皿中，后续进行冷冻保存。在胚胎移植术后 5～6 周，通过超声心动图筛查，根据存在妊娠囊与否诊断临床妊娠情况。

统计分析采用 t 检验，$P<0.05$ 表示有统计学上的显著差异。

3 结果

3.1 新发现

在 2008—2009 年，我们经常观察到患者的胚胎对不同培养基有不同的反应。部分患者的胚胎倾向于在 Global 培养基中优势生长，而一些患者的胚胎倾向于在 P1 培养基中优势生长，一些胚胎在 Global 培养基和 P1 培养基中均生长良好，这意味着胚胎可能对培养基具有良好的选择性（图 7-3）。

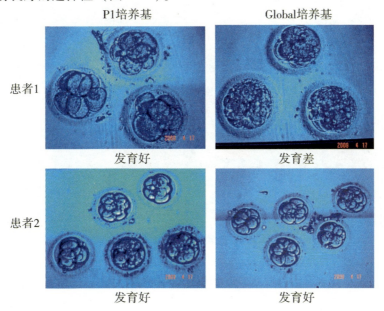

图 7-3 两名患者同一发育时期的胚胎在两种不同培养基中的发育情况

同一天 2 名患者的胚胎被置于两种培养基中。患者 1 的胚胎在 P1 培养基中生长良好（左），但在 Global 培养基中有大量碎片（右）。然而，患者 2 的 10 个胚胎在两种培养基中均生长良好。

3.2 实验验证

为验证我们之前的观察结果，本研究使用了两种不同的商用培养基（P1 培养基和 Global 培养基），共研究了 220 个连续患者周期中 1 850 个正常受精的 2PN 合子，比较第 2 天和第 3 天的卵裂率和优质胚胎比例。结果表明，两种培养基的合子分裂率相同；在第 2 天和第 3 天，Global 培养基似乎产生了略高的优质胚胎比例，但两种培养基之间的差异无统计学意义（$P > 0.05$）（表 7-1 和图 7-4）。当患者的同胞胚胎在两种培养箱中培养时，其卵裂率以及第 2 天和第 3 天的顶级胚胎比例并没有显示出任何显著差异（$P > 0.05$）（图 7-5）。

表 7-1　不同培养基中患者同胞胚胎的发育情况

胚胎级别	发生胚胎数/总胚胎数			
	Medium 培养基		Incubator 培养基	
	Global	P1	Forma	Minc
卵裂	907/930（97.5%[a]）	808/920（98.7%[a]）	992/1025（96.8%[a]）	807/825（97.8%[a]）
第 2 天顶级胚胎	633/845（74.9%[a]）	624/836（74.6%[a]）	730/988（73.9%[a]）	598/800（74.8%[a]）
第 3 天顶级胚胎	564/857（65.8%[a]）	477/768（62.1%[a]）	573/902（63.3%[a]）	478/726（65.8%[a]）

a：两个培养基组之间无显著性差异（$P > 0.05$）。

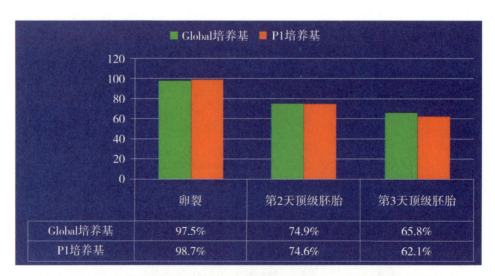

图 7-4　在两种培养基中培养的患者胚胎在卵裂以及第 2 天和第 3 天高质量胚胎方面没有显示出任何显著差异

第 7 章 两种不同类型培养基和两种不同款型培养箱协同作用改善辅助生殖技术妊娠结局

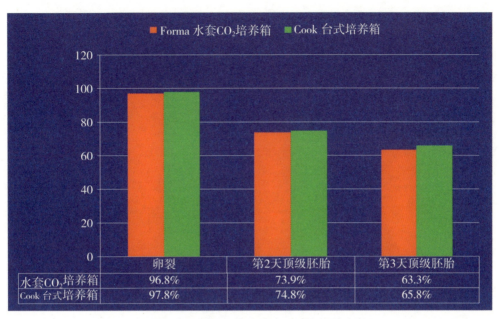

图 7-5 在两种培养箱中培养的患者胚胎在卵裂以及第 2 天和第 3 天高质量胚胎方面没有显示出任何显著差异

然而，当患者同胞胚胎在两种培养基中培养时，一些患者胚胎在 P1 培养基中发育良好，而一些患者胚胎在 Global 培养基中生长良好。这里我们提供了 4 个患者样本，以显示患者胚胎对两种培养基的反应（图 7-6 至图 7-9）。

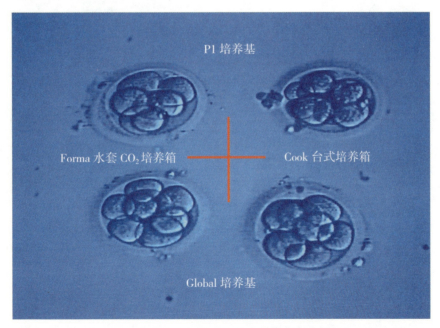

图 7-6 一名 38 岁妇女的 4 个胚胎在两种培养基和两种培养箱中均生长良好
（第 3 天顶级胚胎在同一显微镜下的显示情况）

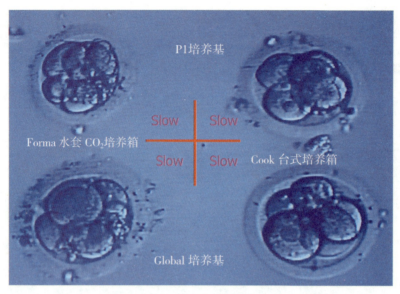

图7-7 一名23岁妇女的4个胚胎在两种培养基和两种培养箱中生长非常差
（第3天顶级胚胎在同一显微镜下的显示情况）

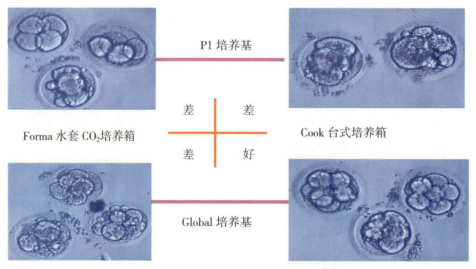

图7-8 一名33岁妇女的8个胚胎在两种培养箱中使用P1培养基，在Forma水套CO_2培养箱中使用Global培养基，结果显示生长均非常差；在Cook台式培养箱的Global培养基中获得了3个优质胚胎

第7章 两种不同类型培养基和两种不同款型培养箱协同作用改善辅助生殖技术妊娠结局

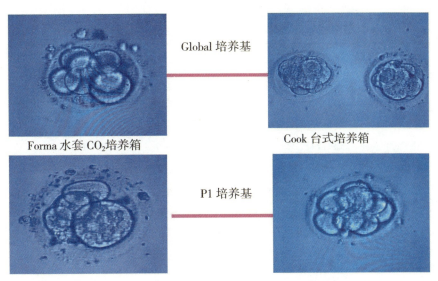

图7-9 一位41岁妇女的4个胚胎在两种培养箱中使用Global培养基，在Cook台式培养箱中使用P1培养基生长均良好，只有1个胚胎在Forma水套CO_2培养箱的P1培养基中质量较差

有些患者胚胎在第2天未被观察，只在第3天进行观察。第2天优质胚胎显示2～6个细胞/5级，第3天优质胚胎显示5～8个细胞/5级。

患者A，38岁，2013年9月30日取回5个卵母细胞，4个受精卵分别在Forma水套CO_2培养箱和Cook台式培养箱中用P1培养基和Global培养基培养。第3天，所有胚胎在各种条件下均表现出良好的质量。

患者B，23岁，2013年10月4日取回13个卵母细胞，4个受精卵分别在Forma水套CO_2培养箱和Cook台式培养箱中用P1培养基和Global培养基培养。第3天，所有胚胎在各种条件下均表现出低质量和缓慢生长。

患者C，33岁，2013年9月30日取回14个卵母细胞，11个合子分别在Forma水套CO_2培养箱和Cook台式培养箱中的P1培养基和Global微滴培养基（每滴培养1个胚胎）中培养。第3天，在Cook台式培养箱的Global培养基中仅获得了3个优质胚胎，其他8个胚胎在其他3种条件下质量较低。

患者D，41岁，2013年10月4日取回5个卵母细胞，5个受精卵分别在Forma水套CO_2培养箱和Cook台式培养箱中的P1培养基和Global培养基中单独培养。第3天，在Forma培养箱的P1培养基中，只有1个胚胎的质量较差，其他4个胚胎的质量较好。

这些结果表明，不同患者的胚胎对不同培养基有不同的反应。为了比较更大量的数据，174名患者的1 875个胚胎被分为4组。第一组有45%（78/174）的患者胚胎在Global培养基或P1培养基中均生长良好；第二组有22%（38/174）的患者胚胎仅在Global培养基中生长良好，而在P1培养基中质量较差；第三组有21%（37/174）的患者胚胎在P1培养基中生长良好，但在Global培养基中生长不良；第四组有12%（21/174）的患者胚胎在P1和Global培养基中均生长不良（表7-2和图7-10）。可以清楚看出一些患者胚胎在Global培养基或P1培养基中生长良好，这表明患者胚胎对于培养基具有选择性。

表7-2　不同培养基中患者同胞胚胎差异发育情况

培养基中的胚胎质量	入组患者/总患者	Global 培养基		P1 培养基	
		胚胎数目	顶级胚胎 $\bar{x} \pm SD$	胚胎数目	顶级胚胎 $\bar{x} \pm SD$
①	78/174（45%）	391/448	87.6 ± 16.30^a	359/425	84.5 ± 16.2^a
②	38/174（22%）	153/190	80.7 ± 22.8^a	67/205	32.8 ± 19.1^b
③	37/174（21%）	51/185	27.7 ± 20.6^a	137/200	68.3 ± 22.5^b
④	21/174（12%）	30/105	28.8 ± 17.7^a	26/120	21.9 ± 20.9^a

a：同一上标表示无显著性差异（$P>0.05$）。b：不同上标表示有显著性差异（$P<0.05$）。
①Global 培养基和 P1 培养基中均发育好；②Global 培养基中发育好，P1 培养基中发育差；③P1 培养基中发育好，Global 培养基中发育差；④Global 培养基和 P1 培养基中均发育差。

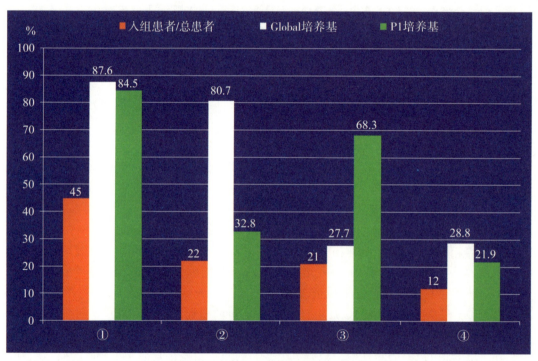

①Global 培养基和 P1 培养基中均发育好；②Global 培养基中发育好，P1 培养基中发育差；③P1 培养基中发育好，Global 培养基中发育差；④Global 培养基和 P1 培养基中均发育差。

图7-10　患者胚胎在两种培养基中的生长情况分布特点

统计结果表明，P1 培养基的妊娠率为 40%（10/25），Global 培养基的妊娠率为 42.5%（9/21）（$P>0.05$）。但是，当两种培养基同时进行胚胎培养时，妊娠率显著增加至 70.1%（122/174）。同时，当两种培养基在两种培养箱中进行胚胎培养时，其妊娠率显著高于单种培养箱（73.2% vs 60%，$P<0.05$）（图7-11）。

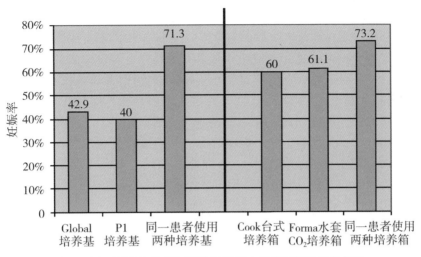

图 7-11　两种培养基和两种培养箱中患者妊娠结局的统计

4　讨论

近 40 年来，ART 已被广泛应用于不孕不育夫妇的治疗，以实现他们生育的梦想。然而，目前试管婴儿成功率仍然保持在 40% 左右的低水平。目前正在通过不断改进和改良体外培养基系统以及创新胚胎选择技术（如时差成像、植入前遗传学诊断和筛查）提高 IVF 的妊娠率。目前已有大量关于不同培养基配方及其对胚胎分裂和胚泡形成的影响的研究[12]。尽管当前商业培养基的组成差异很大，但它们都可很好地支持人类胚胎的体外培养。因此，胚胎培养基的选择取决于胚胎学家的兴趣及其特定工作条件。

在此，我们报告了一项新的观察结果：在临床 IVF-ET 中，患者的胚胎对培养基的反应存在特异性差异。有些患者的胚胎在 Global 培养基中生长更好，有些患者的胚胎在 P1 培养基中生长更好，有些胚胎在 Global 培养基和 P1 培养基中都生长良好，有些患者的胚胎在 P1 培养基和 Global 培养基中都不能很好地生长，这意味着不同的患者胚胎对培养基具有明显的选择性。胚胎培养的目的是获得高质量的胚胎并移植到女性子宫。由于患者胚胎对培养基具有选择性，当将患者的所有胚胎置于单一培养基中培养时，可能所有胚胎质量都很好或很差。如果用单一培养基培养导致患者的所有胚胎质量都较差，则该患者本次 IVF 失败。然而，当胚胎在两种培养基中培养时，有些胚胎在一种培养基中的质量可能很差，但有些胚胎在另一种培养基中的质量可能很好，因此，该患者仍有高质量的胚胎可供移植，以确保增加怀孕机会。

我们的统计结果显示，45% 的患者的胚胎在 Global 培养基或 P1 培养基中均生长良好。因此，无论运用 P1 或 Global 培养基，都有 45% 的患者的胚胎始终生长良好，这是容易获得成功妊娠的群体。另外，大约 12% 的患者的胚胎在 P1 或 Global 培养基中都不能生长良好，这组患者的胚胎无论如何培养都很难致妊娠成功，因为他们无法获得优质胚胎进行成功移植，这可能是由于患者本身的卵母细胞质量或精子质量较差所致。其余约 43% 的患者的胚胎表现出真正地对培养基具有选择性，22% 的患者胚胎仅在 P1 培养基中生长良好但在 Global 培养基中质量较差，而 21% 的患者胚胎在 Global 培养基中生长良好但在 P1 培养基中生长较差。因此，通过选择培养基，我们可以从这 43% 的患者群体中获得高质量的胚胎。因此，在目前的 IVF 技术下，IVF 成功率最高可达到 88%（45%+43%=88%）。按照移植胚胎妇女的不同年龄进行分组，表 7-3 列出了各组在两种培养基和两种培养箱中的妊娠率。这种非常高的妊娠率导致 20.7% 的双胞胎和 3.74% 的三胞胎出生，表明两种培养基确实增加了移植胚胎植入的机会，改善了临床结局，但在临床实践中，移植胚胎的数量应相应减少。

表 7-3　用两种培养基和两种培养箱进行胚胎培养和混合胚胎移植的妊娠结果

患者年龄	移植胚胎数目	妊娠数目
<28	1.98（1～2）	20/23（86.96%）
28～34	2.64（1～3）	50/67（74.63%）
35～27	2.94（2～4）	24/33（72.72%）
38～40	3.12（1～4）	21/32（65.63%）
>40	3.81（2～4）	9/21（42.86%）

从两种培养基中选择优质胚胎移植，可显著改善 IVF 临床结局。Wirleitner 等[17]曾报道过一个有趣的观察结果，即移植 2 个分别来自不同培养基的胚胎，会导致双胞胎妊娠率显著提高。我们的研究表明，使用两种不同培养基培养同一患者胚胎可获得约 71% 的妊娠率。然而，如果使用单一培养基进行培养，只有约 40% 的妊娠率。在一种培养箱中使用两种培养基进行培养可提高 60% 的妊娠率。当使用两种培养基并在两种培养箱中共同培养时，妊娠率可提高到 73%。因此，应用两种培养基和两种培养箱可以显著改善人类 IVF/ICSI 临床妊娠结局。

5　结论

在临床 IVF 实践中，患者对商用培养基的特异性反应似乎起着重要作用，为确保每个患者都有足够的高质量胚胎用于移植，建议每个患者的胚胎培养应用两种不同类型的培养基和两种不同类型的培养箱结合培养。个别患者的胚胎对培养基和培养箱的良好反应表明，在 IVF 临床实践中，使用两种培养基和两种培养箱同时进行胚胎培养可以显著提高 IVF/ICSI 妊娠率。

参考文献

[1] BRACHETM A. Recherches sur la de" terminisme he're'ditaire de l'oeuf des mammife'res. De'veloppement in vitro de jeunes ve'sicules blastodermiques de lapin [M]. Archives de Biologie (lie'ge). 1913, 28: 423-426.

[2] BIGGERS J D. IVF and embryo transfer: historical origin and development [J]. Fertility magazine. 2012, 25 (2): 118-127.

[3] WHITTEN W K. Culture of tubal mouse ova [J]. Nature, 1956, 177 (4498): 96.

[4] QUINN P, KERIN J F, WARNES G M. Improved pregnancy rate in human in vitro fertilization with the use of a medium based on the composition of human tubal fluid [J]. Fertility and sterility, 1985, 44 (4): 493-498.

[5] BIGGERS J D. Thoughts on embryo culture conditions [J]. Reproductive biomedicine online, 2002, 4 Suppl 1: 30-38.

[6] BIGGERS J D. History of KSOM, a single medium for embryo culture [J]. Fertility World. 2005, 3: 4-7.

[7] RIEGER D. A single medium can support development of human embryos to the blastocyst stage [J]. Fertility World. 2005, 3: 24-27.

[8] EDWARDS R G. Test-tube babies, 1981 [J]. Nature, 1981, 293 (5830): 253-256.

[9] GARDNER D K, LANE M. Embryo culture systems [M]. 2nd ed. USA: CRC Press LLC, 2000.

[10] FONG C Y, BONGSO A. Comparison of human blastulation rates and total cell number in sequential culture media with and without co-culture [J]. Human reproduction, 1998, 14 (3): 774-781.

[11] MORBECK D E, BAUMANN N A, OGLESBEE D. Composition of single-step media used for human embryo culture [J]. Fertility and sterility, 2017, 107 (4): 1055-1060.

[12] MORBECK D E, KRISHER R L, HERRICK J R, et al. Composition of commercial media used for human embryo culture [J]. Fertility and sterility, 2014, 102 (3): 759-766.

[13] AOKI V W, WILCOX A L, PETERSON C M, et al. Comparison of four media types during 3-day human IVF embryo culture [J]. Reproductive biomedicine online, 2005, 10 (5): 600-606.

[14] CHRONOPOULOU E, HARPER J C. IVF culture media: past, present and future [J]. Human reproduction update, 2015, 21 (1): 39-55.

[15] MANTIKOU E, YOUSSEF M A F M, VAN WELY M, et al. Embryo culture media and IVF/ICSI success rates: a systematic review [J]. Human reproduction update, 2013, 19 (3): 210-220.

[16] SWAIN J E. Optimal human embryo culture [J]. Seminars in reproductive medicine, 2015, 33 (2): 103-117.

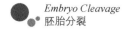

[17] WIRLEITNER B, VANDERZWALMEN P, STECHER A, et al. Individual demands of human embryos on IVF culture medium: influence on blastocyst development and pregnancy outcome [J]. Reproductive biomedicine online, 2010, 21 (6): 776 – 782.

(Bin Wu, Jinzhou Qin, Suzhen Lu, Linda Wu and Timothy J. Gelety)